GOLDEN YEARS DEEP BREATHS

OXYGEN'S POWER FOR SENIORS

JIM PHILLIPS

TABLE OF CONTENTS

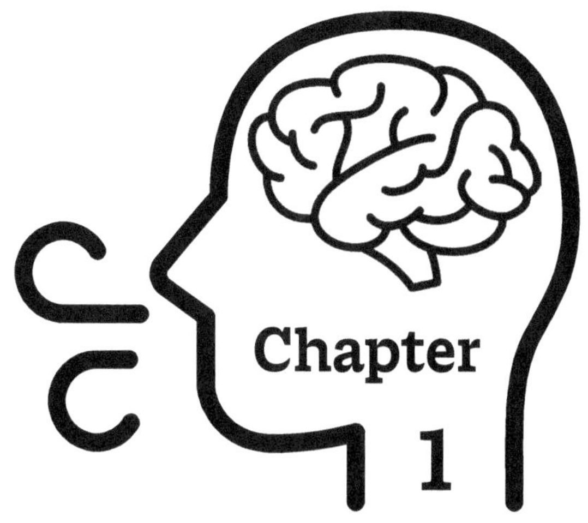

INTRODUCTION TO BREATHING AND AGING

With a relaxed breath, let your mind wander to a peaceful bamboo sanctuary, where the gentle ripple of water and the soothing chorus of birds instill a sense of serenity, guiding you into a mindful space, prepared to absorb the life-affirming lessons of breath and awareness in this chapter.

Welcome to "Golden Years, Deep Breaths: Oxygen's Power for Seniors," a guide dedicated to enhancing the lives of seniors through the simple yet profound practice of breathing exercises. This book is the culmination of years of personal experience and a deep appreciation for the transformative benefits that daily breathing exercises can offer, especially as we age. The author's approach is grounded in the belief that the wisdom of ancient yoga practices should be shared in a way that resonates with our modern lives and be specifically geared for the Golden Years. Through this work, the author aims to make these beneficial practices more accessible, helping readers to unlock their potential for improved health and increased vitality.

In this book, we want to assure you that you don't need to be daunted by the terminology or associations with practices like Yoga breathing exercises or foreign words that describe these techniques. Instead, we focus on breathing exercises that work, which have been developed, practiced, and tested for thousands of years. Our goal is straightforward: to emphasize the incredible power and benefits of daily breathing exercises, as well as the profound impact of oxygen on our overall well-being.

As we age, our bodies, including our respiratory systems, undergo significant changes that can affect our quality of life. These changes are often accepted as inevitable aspects of aging. However, we believe that with the right knowledge and practices, seniors can maintain and even improve their respiratory health, enhancing their overall well-being in their golden years.

Through this book, we aim to empower you, our cherished readers, with practical insights and user-friendly techniques that are tailored to address the unique needs of seniors. Our hope is that you will discover the transformative potential of conscious breathing and experience the positive impact it can have on your health and vitality as you navigate the golden years of life.

Additionally, we believe that educating ourselves is a beneficial power in and of itself. Therefore, this book also aims to provide you with a comprehensive education on all aspects of breathing. We want you to not only benefit from the exercises and practices but also understand the underlying science and principles. Informed and empowered, you'll be equipped to make the most of the remarkable power of your own breath, enhancing your well-being at any stage of life.

Breathing, an act so fundamental to life, holds the key to enhanced well-being, and this book serves as your comprehensive guide to unlocking these benefits. We delve into the science of breathing and aging, present effective breathing exercises, and explain how these can positively impact your health. Whether you're looking to boost your energy levels, improve lung function, or simply find a new way to relax and de-stress, the practices detailed here are tailored to meet these needs.

Target Audience: "Golden Years, Deep Breaths" is crafted for a wide audience, with a primary focus on seniors who wish to explore the rejuvenating power of breathing exercises. However, the content is equally relevant and accessible to caregivers, family members, and healthcare professionals who support senior health and well-being. It is also an invaluable resource for anyone interested in learning about the aging process and how mindful breathing can mitigate its effects.

"The Golden Years" is, of course, a term we all commonly used to refer to the period of life typically associated with retirement and senior citizenship. It is supposed to signify a phase in one's life characterized by a combination of factors, including the attainment of a certain age, the culmination of a career, and the transition into a more leisurely and reflective lifestyle. These years are often viewed as a time of well-deserved relaxation, self-discovery, and the pursuit of personal interests and passions that may have been put on hold during earlier stages of life. And we hope that is the case for everyone.

While "The Golden Years" are often seen as a time of retirement from formal employment, they are also an opportunity for continued growth, learning, and enjoying the fruits of one's labor. It's a period when individuals may spend more time with family, travel, explore new hobbies, and reflect on their life experiences. These years, typically associated with the later stages of life, offer the freedom and opportunity to make the most of one's time and experiences.

The journey of aging is indeed unique for everyone, but there are common threads that connect us all. This book aims to address these universal aspects of aging, providing guidance rooted in both scientific knowledge and empathy. Importantly, it's crucial to recognize that aging is a continuous process that touches every stage of life. Therefore, the benefits of practicing these breathing exercises extend to individuals of all ages.

Furthermore, many seniors may undergo surgeries along their aging journey, where the importance of adequate oxygen levels becomes crucial both in preparing for surgery and facilitating post-surgery recovery. This underscores the significance of understanding and harnessing the power of oxygen, as exemplified in the science behind hyperbaric therapy, a medical treatment that involves breathing pure oxygen in a pressurized chamber, often used to promote healing and treat various medical conditions as advised by with qualified healthcare professionals to determine its suitability for their specific needs and conditions.

Whether you're a senior who is seeking ways to enhance your physical and mental well-being, a caregiver looking for methods to support your loved ones, or simply someone interested in the art of breathing for better health, this book is your companion on a journey towards improved respiratory health and overall well-being throughout life's stages.

In the chapters that follow, we will delve into the transformative power of conscious breathing, guiding you through a journey of discovery, wellness, and empowerment. We want to remind you that oxygen is not just a substance; it's a necessity for life itself. Through the pages of this book, you'll learn how to nourish your body with this life-giving element, unlocking its incredible potential to enhance your health and vitality.

Welcome to a journey of breath, a journey to a better, healthier you. Regardless of where you are on the path of life, the simple act of breathing consciously can lead to profound changes in your well-being and overall quality of life.

The Importance of Lung Health in Seniors

As we age, our bodies undergo various changes, and the respiratory system is no exception. Understanding these changes is crucial in recognizing the importance of maintaining lung health during our senior years.

Changes in Respiratory System with Age: One of the most significant changes that occur in the respiratory system as we age is the reduction in lung capacity. This decrease can be attributed to several factors. Firstly, the diaphragm muscles, which play a vital role in the breathing process, become weaker, reducing their efficiency in expanding and contracting the lungs. Additionally, the ribcage and spine may undergo structural changes due to osteoporosis or other age-related conditions, limiting the ability of the chest to expand fully during inhalation.

Furthermore, the alveoli, tiny air sacs in the lungs where oxygen and carbon dioxide are exchanged, lose some of their elasticity. This loss leads to less efficient gas exchange, meaning less oxygen can enter the bloodstream and fewer waste gases can be expelled with each breath. These changes, while natural, can significantly impact a senior's respiratory efficiency and overall health.

Challenges Faced by Seniors: Due to these changes, seniors often face several respiratory challenges. Shortness of breath, or dyspnea, is a common issue. It can occur even during light activities that were previously manageable, such as walking or climbing stairs. This shortness of breath is not just uncomfortable; it can lead to a reduction in physical activity, further exacerbating health issues.

Another major challenge is the increased susceptibility to respiratory illnesses. As the immune system weakens with age, the body's ability to fight off infections like influenza or pneumonia diminishes. These illnesses can have a more severe impact on seniors, often leading to prolonged recovery times and, in some cases, serious complications.

Recognizing these challenges is the first step in addressing them. By understanding how the respiratory system changes with age, seniors and their caregivers can take proactive measures to maintain lung health. This may include engaging in specific breathing exercises, making lifestyle changes, and staying vigilant about respiratory health, especially during cold and flu season. The subsequent chapters of this book delve deeper into practical strategies and exercises to strengthen the respiratory system, enhance lung capacity, and improve overall respiratory health in seniors. This proactive approach is key to enjoying a healthier, more active lifestyle in the golden years.

The Role of Breathing Exercises

In the context of aging and respiratory health, breathing exercises emerge as a powerful, yet often underutilized, tool. These exercises offer a range of benefits that are particularly significant for seniors, touching upon various aspects of their health and well-being.

Benefits of Breathing Exercises: The primary benefit of breathing exercises for seniors is the improvement of lung function. Regular practice helps strengthen the respiratory muscles, making them more efficient in their function. This improvement in muscle strength can lead to increased lung capacity, allowing more air to fill the lungs, thereby enhancing the oxygenation process. Enhanced oxygenation ensures that vital organs and tissues receive an adequate supply of oxygen, which is crucial for maintaining overall health and vitality.

Another significant benefit is the reduction of stress. Breathing exercises, particularly those that emphasize slow and deep breathing, activate the body's parasympathetic nervous system. This activation induces a state of relaxation, reducing stress hormone levels, and mitigating the effects of stress on the body. For seniors, this is especially beneficial, as stress can exacerbate existing health conditions and impede the body's natural healing processes.

In addition to improving lung function and reducing stress, these exercises also contribute to overall health enhancement. They can aid in regulating blood pressure, improving sleep quality, enhancing digestion, and boosting immune function. The holistic impact of breathing exercises on health can significantly enhance the quality of life for seniors, making daily activities more manageable and enjoyable.

Scientific Evidence: The effectiveness of breathing exercises is not just anecdotal but is also backed by scientific research. Studies have shown that practices like diaphragmatic breathing and paced respiration can have measurable impacts on respiratory function, mental health, and overall well-being in older adults. For instance, a study published in the Journal of Cardiopulmonary Rehabilitation and Prevention found that lung function, as measured by factors like forced expiratory volume, showed significant improvement in older adults who engaged in regular breathing exercises.

Further, research in the field of psychoneuroimmunology has established a link between stress reduction techniques, such as deep breathing exercises, and improved immune response. This link is particularly relevant for seniors, as a robust immune system is crucial for maintaining health and preventing illness.

In conclusion, breathing exercises offer a range of benefits that are particularly advantageous for seniors. They serve as a simple, yet effective, tool for improving lung function, reducing stress, and enhancing overall health. The subsequent chapters of this book will guide you through various breathing exercises, each designed to target specific aspects of respiratory and overall health, backed by scientific understanding and evidence.

Understanding the Basics of Breathing

Grasping the fundamentals of how we breathe is key to appreciating the importance of breathing exercises, especially for seniors. This understanding begins with the anatomy of breathing and extends to the crucial role oxygen plays in maintaining cellular health and overall vitality.

Anatomy of Breathing: Breathing is a complex yet beautifully orchestrated process involving several key organs, primarily the lungs and the diaphragm. The lungs, a pair of spongy, air-filled organs located on either side of the chest, are the central players in the respiratory system. When you inhale, air travels through your nose or mouth, down the trachea, and into the bronchial tubes within the lungs. These tubes branch out into smaller tubes, ending in clusters of tiny air sacs called alveoli.

The diaphragm, a dome-shaped muscle located below the lungs, plays a pivotal role in breathing. As you inhale, the diaphragm contracts and flattens, creating a vacuum that pulls air into the lungs. As the lungs expand, oxygen from the air passes through the walls of the alveoli and into the bloodstream. Simultaneously, carbon dioxide, a waste product of metabolism, moves from the blood into the alveoli to be exhaled. This exchange of gases is fundamental to the respiratory process and is essential for maintaining the body's vital functions.

Oxygen's Role in the Body: Oxygen is critical for life. Every cell in the body requires oxygen to perform cellular respiration, a process that converts nutrients from food into energy. This energy is essential for every bodily function, from moving muscles to thinking thoughts. Without adequate oxygen, cells cannot produce enough energy, leading to fatigue and diminished function.

Beyond energy production, oxygen plays a vital role in maintaining cognitive functions. The brain, which consumes about 20% of the body's oxygen supply, relies heavily on this element to maintain its operations. Adequate oxygenation ensures that the brain can function optimally, supporting everything from memory and concentration to decision-making processes.

For seniors, maintaining efficient breathing and ensuring adequate oxygen supply is crucial. Age-related changes can impact the efficiency of the respiratory system, but through targeted breathing exercises, it's possible to enhance lung capacity and oxygenation. This, in turn, can lead to improvements in energy levels, cognitive function, and overall well-being, making the golden years not just more manageable but also more enjoyable. The upcoming chapters will guide you through various breathing techniques to maximize these benefits, helping you to breathe better and live better.

Addressing Common Misconceptions

When it comes to aging and respiratory health, there are numerous myths that can create unnecessary barriers for seniors. Understanding and dispelling these myths is crucial in empowering seniors to take proactive steps towards maintaining and improving their respiratory health.

Myths About Aging and Breathing: One prevalent myth is that declining lung function is an inevitable part of aging that cannot be mitigated. While it's true that lung capacity naturally decreases with age, this decline can be significantly slowed down with proper care and exercise. Research has shown that regular, targeted breathing exercises can enhance lung capacity, improve the efficiency of the respiratory muscles, and even increase the body's oxygen uptake. Therefore, seniors should be reassured that their efforts towards maintaining respiratory health are not in vain and can lead to substantial improvements in their quality of life.

Another common misconception is that seniors with existing respiratory conditions or those who have never engaged in physical activities cannot benefit from breathing exercises. This is far from the truth. In fact, breathing exercises are highly adaptable and can be tailored to fit individuals with various health conditions and fitness levels. Even gentle, low impact breathing techniques can yield significant benefits, including better oxygenation, stress reduction, and enhanced lung function.

Encouragement for Beginners: For seniors who are new to breathing exercises, it's important to emphasize that these practices are not only accessible but also highly beneficial, regardless of their current health status or fitness level. Breathing exercises do not require any special equipment or a high degree of physical exertion, making them an ideal activity for seniors.

Starting with simple techniques such as diaphragmatic breathing or paced breathing can introduce seniors to the practice in a comfortable and manageable way. These exercises can be performed anywhere, whether sitting in a chair, lying in bed, or standing. The key is to begin slowly, listen to one's body, and gradually increase the duration and intensity of the exercises as comfort and ability improve.

Encouragement and reassurance are vital. Seniors should be reminded that making small, consistent efforts in practicing breathing exercises can lead to noticeable improvements in their respiratory health, overall energy levels, and mental clarity. With patience and persistence, breathing exercises can become a valuable and enjoyable part of their daily routine, contributing significantly to their health and well-being in their golden years.

Personal Stories and Testimonials: Incorporated throughout the book are heartening testimonials from seniors who have embraced these breathing exercises and witnessed remarkable improvements in their lives.

For instance, Jim, the author of this book, has for years used the benefits of alternate nostril breathing as a solution for clearing his sinuses during the night before he wakes up. Jim attests that this practice not only helps him breathe more freely but also promotes restful sleep, making his mornings more rejuvenating and his days more vibrant. He, also, has been using diaphragmatic breathing for over 55 years into his daily routine not only to improve his lung capacity but also significantly reduced stress levels. And, John, a 72-year-old retiree, shares how incorporating diaphragmatic breathing into his daily routine has not only improved his lung capacity but also significantly reduced his stress levels. Similarly, 68-year-old Maria recounts how yoga breathing practices have enhanced her focus and brought a newfound sense of calm to her life.

These stories are not just narratives; they are testaments from real, everyday life to the transformative power of regular breathing exercises. They serve as inspiration and motivation, showcasing the tangible benefits that can be achieved regardless of age or current fitness level.

As we progress through each chapter, these insights and practices will equip you with the knowledge and tools needed to enhance your respiratory health and overall well-being. Welcome to a journey of discovery, empowerment, and rejuvenation.

Conclusion and Invitation to Begin: As we reach the conclusion of this introductory chapter, it's time to extend a heartfelt invitation for you to embark on this transformative journey. "Golden Years, Deep Breaths: Oxygen's Power for Seniors" is more than just a guide; it's a pathway to enhanced health and well-being, tailored specifically for the golden years of life.

Encouragement to Start the Journey: I want to encourage you, the reader, to take the first step with optimism and curiosity. Whether you are a senior seeking to improve your respiratory health, a caregiver looking for ways to support your loved one, or simply someone interested in the art of breathing for better health, this book offers you a treasure trove of insights and practical techniques. The journey into breathing exercises is not just about enhancing lung capacity or oxygen intake; it's a journey towards a more fulfilled, energized, and balanced life.

The practices detailed in this book are more than mere exercises; they are steppingstones to a renewed sense of vitality and tranquility. Embarking on this journey doesn't require drastic changes or overwhelming efforts. It starts with small, consistent steps – a few minutes a day dedicated to the practices outlined in these chapters. As you progress, you'll discover the remarkable ability of the body to respond, adapt, and thrive, even in the later stages of life.

Setting Expectations: It's important to approach this journey with realistic expectations. The benefits of breathing exercises don't manifest overnight but unfold gradually over time. You may notice initial improvements in your breathing, a sense of calm, or a boost in energy levels. Over time, these changes can become more pronounced, leading to significant improvements in your respiratory health, mental clarity, and overall well-being.

Remember, everyone's experience is unique, and progress may vary. Be patient with yourself and acknowledge every small victory along the way. The key to success lies in regular practice and a commitment to incorporating these exercises into your daily routine.

As you turn the pages of this book and begin to practice the exercises, know that you are taking a powerful step towards a healthier, more vibrant version of yourself. Welcome to a journey of discovery, empowerment, and renewal. Let's breathe new life into your golden years!

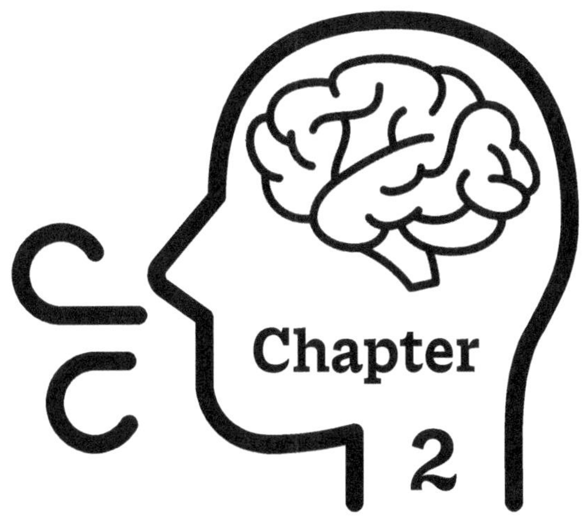

THE SCIENCE OF BREATH
AND OXYGEN

With a relaxed breath, let your mind wander to a peaceful bamboo sanctuary, where the gentle ripple of water and the soothing chorus of birds instill a sense of serenity, guiding you into a mindful space, prepared to absorb the life-affirming lessons of breath and awareness in this chapter.

In this chapter, we delve into the fascinating world of the science behind breathing and the indispensable role of oxygen in our bodies. This exploration is crucial, particularly for seniors, as understanding these aspects can be transformative in managing and enhancing their overall health and well-being.

Importance of Understanding Breathing: Why is it essential for seniors to understand the mechanics of breathing? As we age, our bodies undergo numerous changes, and the respiratory system is no exception. A clear understanding of how breathing works provides valuable insights into why certain respiratory issues may arise and how they can be effectively managed or mitigated. Moreover, with age, the efficiency of our breathing process often diminishes. By comprehending the mechanics of breathing, seniors can proactively engage in practices that optimize their respiratory function, thereby enhancing their oxygen intake and overall vitality.

The act of breathing is not just a simple in-and-out movement of air; it's a complex process involving the lungs, diaphragm, and a host of other physiological elements. A deeper understanding of this process illuminates the pathways to maintaining and improving respiratory health, especially as one navigates the later stages of life.

Goal of the Chapter: The objective of this chapter is to provide a thorough and accessible overview of the physiological aspects of breathing. We will explore how the respiratory system functions, the process of gas exchange, and the mechanics involved in each breath we take. Furthermore, this chapter will highlight the critical role oxygen plays in our bodies, from supporting cellular function to maintaining cognitive health.

By the end of this chapter, readers will have a comprehensive understanding of the science of breathing and oxygenation. This knowledge is not merely academic; it's practical and empowering. It lays the foundation for implementing effective breathing exercises and lifestyle changes that can profoundly impact seniors' respiratory health and overall quality of life. Let's embark on this educational journey together, exploring the science of breath and the life-sustaining power of oxygen.

Understanding the Respiratory System: Gaining an understanding of the respiratory system is fundamental in appreciating how our bodies function and the vital role breathing plays in our overall health. This system, intricate and elegantly designed, ensures that every cell in our body receives the oxygen it needs to function properly.

Basic Anatomy of the Respiratory System: At the core of the respiratory system are the lungs, two sponge-like, air-filled organs situated within the chest cavity. The lungs' primary function is to facilitate the exchange of gases - taking in oxygen and expelling carbon dioxide. Air enters the body through the nose or mouth, travels down the trachea (windpipe), and reaches the lungs via a network of bronchi that branch out into smaller tubes called bronchioles, finally ending in tiny sacs known as alveoli. It is in these alveoli where the critical exchange of oxygen and carbon dioxide occurs.

The diaphragm, a dome-shaped muscle located just below the lungs, plays a pivotal role in the breathing process. As the main muscle responsible for breathing, it contracts and flattens when you inhale, creating a vacuum that draws air into the lungs.

The Breathing Process: Inhalation begins with the contraction of the diaphragm, which expands the chest cavity and decreases the pressure inside the lungs compared to the outside atmosphere, causing air to flow in. Simultaneously, the muscles between the ribs, known as the intercostal muscles, also contract, further expanding the chest cavity.

Exhalation is largely a passive process during rest, resulting from the relaxation of the diaphragm and intercostal muscles. This relaxation causes the chest cavity to decrease in size, increasing the pressure in the lungs and pushing air out. During vigorous activities, exhalation becomes an active process where the abdominal muscles contract to push the diaphragm up more forcefully, expelling air more rapidly.

Understanding these components and their functions in the respiratory process is crucial, especially for seniors. It underscores the importance of maintaining respiratory health and offers insight into how specific breathing exercises can enhance lung efficiency, contributing significantly to overall well-being.

Oxygen and the Body: Oxygen plays a fundamental role in sustaining life, serving as a crucial element for cellular function, energy production, and maintaining organ health. Its significance becomes even more pronounced as we age, making an understanding of its functions and transportation within the body essential.

Role of Oxygen in the Body: Every cell in the human body requires oxygen to perform aerobic respiration, a process that converts glucose and oxygen into energy, carbon dioxide, and water. This energy, known as ATP (adenosine triphosphate), is vital for all bodily functions, from muscle contractions and brain activity to the maintenance of organ systems. Oxygen is also integral in various metabolic processes and plays a role in immune function, helping to fight off infections and facilitate healing.

Oxygen Transportation: Oxygen transportation in the body is an efficient process, primarily facilitated by the circulatory system.

When we inhale, oxygen enters the lungs and diffuses through the walls of the alveoli into the surrounding capillaries. Here, it binds to hemoglobin, a protein found in red blood cells. Hemoglobin is specially designed to carry oxygen; each molecule can bind up to four oxygen molecules, efficiently transporting them through the bloodstream to various tissues and organs. Once hemoglobin reaches body tissues, it releases oxygen, allowing it to diffuse into cells for use in metabolic processes.

Effects of Aging on Oxygen Utilization: As we age, several changes occur in the body that can affect its ability to utilize oxygen efficiently. The efficiency of respiratory muscles, lung capacity, and the strength of the diaphragm can all diminish, potentially leading to reduced oxygen intake. Additionally, age-related changes in the cardiovascular system, such as reduced heart function and arterial stiffness, can impede the effective transportation of oxygen-rich blood. These factors combined can lead to decreased oxygenation of tissues and organs, which may impact energy levels, cognitive function, and overall health.

Understanding the role of oxygen in the body and how its utilization changes with age is vital. It underscores the importance of practices like breathing exercises, which can help mitigate some of these age-related changes by enhancing lung capacity and promoting more efficient oxygen uptake.

The Science Behind Breathing Exercises

Breathing exercises, particularly deep breathing, are more than just a relaxation technique; they have profound physiological benefits backed by science. Understanding these benefits can motivate seniors to incorporate these exercises into their daily routines, enhancing their overall health and well-being.

Physiological Benefits of Deep Breathing: Deep breathing, characterized by slow and deliberate inhalation and exhalation, has several physiological benefits. Firstly, it increases oxygen intake. By taking deeper breaths, more air is drawn into the lungs, increasing the oxygen supplied to the alveoli and, consequently, to the blood. This enhanced oxygenation supports cellular functions and energy production throughout the body.

Improved lung function is another significant benefit. Deep breathing exercises can help strengthen the respiratory muscles, making them more efficient. This efficiency can improve lung capacity, which tends to decline with age, and assist in clearing the airways, reducing the likelihood of respiratory infections.

Furthermore, deep breathing can positively impact blood circulation. The act of deep breathing creates a pressure gradient in the chest cavity, which assists the return of blood to the heart. Enhanced circulation ensures that oxygen and nutrients are effectively distributed throughout the body, supporting organ function, and aiding in waste removal.

Impact on the Nervous System: Breathing exercises, particularly those focused on deep and rhythmic breathing, have a significant impact on the autonomic nervous system (ANS), which controls the body's involuntary functions, including heart rate and digestion. These exercises can stimulate the parasympathetic nervous system, often referred to as the "rest and digest" system. Activation of the parasympathetic nervous system induces a state of calm and relaxation, reducing stress hormone levels and alleviating symptoms of anxiety.

The effects on the ANS also include a reduction in heart rate and lower blood pressure, further enhancing relaxation and stress relief. This relaxation response can be particularly beneficial for seniors who experience heightened stress levels, which can exacerbate health issues and impede the body's natural healing processes.

In summary, the science behind breathing exercises reveals their capacity to significantly improve physical health by increasing oxygen intake, enhancing lung function, improving circulation, and positively impacting the nervous system. These benefits collectively contribute to reduced stress levels and a heightened sense of relaxation and well-being, making breathing exercises an invaluable tool for seniors.

The Role of Oxygen in Disease Prevention and Management

Oxygen, vital for life and central to numerous bodily functions, plays a significant role in both the prevention and management of various health conditions, particularly those common in seniors. Understanding this role can empower individuals to adopt practices that enhance oxygenation, thereby improving their health and quality of life.

Preventing Respiratory Issues: Effective breathing techniques are crucial in preventing respiratory problems, a concern particularly prevalent among seniors. Deep and controlled breathing exercises can strengthen the respiratory muscles, increase lung capacity, and improve the efficiency of the respiratory system. This enhancement in respiratory function is key in preventing conditions such as chronic bronchitis and pneumonia, which are more common in older adults.

Additionally, regular practice of breathing exercises can help clear the airways, reducing the risk of infections and complications associated with mucus build-up. By improving overall lung function and respiratory health, these exercises serve as a proactive measure in maintaining respiratory wellness and preventing the onset or exacerbation of respiratory issues in seniors.

Managing Chronic Conditions: For seniors dealing with chronic conditions such as Chronic Obstructive Pulmonary Disease (COPD) and heart disease, improved oxygenation through effective breathing practices can be particularly beneficial. In COPD, for example, where the airflow is obstructed, breathing exercises can aid in better air exchange, helping patients manage symptoms and enhance their quality of life.

In the case of heart disease, efficient oxygenation is crucial as it ensures that the heart receives the oxygen-rich blood it needs for optimal function. Practices that enhance lung capacity and oxygen uptake can therefore play a supportive role in managing heart conditions, particularly where oxygen transport and utilization are compromised.

Overall, the role of oxygen in disease prevention and management cannot be overstated. By improving oxygenation through effective breathing techniques, seniors can not only help prevent respiratory issues but also actively manage chronic conditions, contributing significantly to better health outcomes and an enhanced sense of well-being.

Breathing and Cognitive Function

The relationship between oxygen levels and cognitive function is a critical area of interest, particularly for seniors. Oxygen is not only essential for physical health but also plays a pivotal role in maintaining and enhancing cognitive abilities, including memory and concentration.

Oxygen and Brain Health: The brain, which accounts for only about 2% of a person's body weight, consumes roughly 20% of the body's oxygen supply. This high demand underscores the importance of oxygen for brain health. Adequate oxygenation is crucial for the brain's optimal functioning, as it fuels brain cells and helps in the maintenance and repair of neurons. Improved oxygen levels can enhance cognitive functions such as memory, focus, problem-solving abilities, and concentration.

Conversely, reduced oxygen levels can have a detrimental impact on these functions. In seniors, where the risk of decreased oxygen saturation is higher due to various factors like reduced lung capacity and efficiency, maintaining adequate oxygen levels becomes even more crucial. Engaging in breathing exercises that enhance oxygen intake can, therefore, have a positive impact on maintaining and improving cognitive functions in older adults.

Studies and Research: Several scientific studies have highlighted the benefits of improved oxygenation on brain health. For instance, research published in the Journal of the American Geriatrics Society found that higher oxygen saturation levels were associated with better performance in cognitive tests among seniors. Another study in the Journal of Cognitive Neuroscience reported that increased oxygen intake, facilitated by deep breathing exercises, was linked to improved reaction times and accuracy in cognitive tasks.

These findings suggest that practices that enhance oxygenation – like deep breathing exercises – can be beneficial in maintaining and improving cognitive functions in seniors. Not only do these exercises support physical health, but they also contribute to preserving mental acuity, memory, and concentration, which are vital for an independent and fulfilling life in the later years.

Practical Tips for Improving Oxygenation

Enhancing oxygenation is not solely about engaging in specific exercises; it also involves adopting daily habits that support respiratory health. Simple lifestyle changes can significantly impact the body's ability to utilize oxygen efficiently, particularly important for seniors looking to maintain their vitality and overall health.

Daily Habits: Maintain a Healthy Diet: A balanced diet rich in antioxidants can help reduce inflammation in the body, including the lungs, and improve respiratory health. Foods high in antioxidants, such as fruits, vegetables, nuts, and seeds, should be staples in your diet. Omega-3 fatty acids, found in fish and flaxseeds, are also beneficial as they can reduce inflammation in the respiratory system, enhancing oxygenation.

Stay Hydrated: Adequate hydration is crucial for maintaining the health of the mucosal linings in the lungs and airways. Proper hydration ensures these linings can effectively trap and clear out irritants and pathogens. Aim for at least 8 glasses of water a day, more if you're physically active or live in a hot climate.

Quit Smoking: Smoking is one of the most damaging habits for lung health. It impairs lung function and reduces oxygen levels in the body. Quitting smoking can significantly improve lung capacity and efficiency, enhancing oxygenation and overall health.

Simple Exercises for Better Breathing:

Diaphragmatic Breathing: This involves breathing deeply into the lungs, allowing the diaphragm to descend and the abdomen to expand. Practice by lying on your back with one hand on your belly and the other on your chest. Breathe in deeply through your nose, feeling your belly rise more than your chest.

Pursed-Lip Breathing: Inhale slowly through the nose, then exhale gently through pursed lips, as if blowing out a candle. This technique helps control the pace of breathing, making each breath more efficient.

4-7-8 Breathing: Breathe in quietly through your nose for 4 seconds, hold the breath for 7 seconds, and exhale forcefully through your mouth for 8 seconds. This exercise is known to promote relaxation and improve oxygenation.

Incorporating these tips and exercises into your daily routine can lead to improved oxygen levels and better respiratory health. Remember, consistency is key – regular practice and adherence to these lifestyle changes can yield significant health benefits over time.

Myths and Facts About Oxygen Therapy

Oxygen therapy, a treatment that provides extra oxygen to support the respiratory system, is an important topic to understand, particularly when discussing respiratory health in seniors. However, there are several myths and misconceptions surrounding its use and purpose.

Understanding Oxygen Therapy: Oxygen therapy involves administering oxygen at concentrations higher than that in ambient air to treat or prevent low blood oxygen levels. It's commonly used in clinical settings but can also be prescribed for home use, especially for individuals with chronic respiratory conditions such as COPD, pulmonary fibrosis, or severe heart conditions. The therapy can be delivered through nasal tubes, face masks, or more advanced devices like ventilators, depending on the patient's needs and the severity of their condition.

Dispelling Myths

Myth: Oxygen Therapy is Only for the Critically Ill: While it is often used in critical care, oxygen therapy is also prescribed for patients with chronic respiratory conditions to use at home, aiding in their daily living and improving quality of life.

Myth: It's Addictive and Can Make Your Lungs Lazy: There's a common misconception that using supplemental oxygen can make the body or lungs dependent on it or 'lazy.' However, oxygen therapy is prescribed to ensure that individuals with compromised lung function receive adequate oxygenation. It does not cause physical dependence, nor does it reduce the lungs' ability to function on their own.

Myth: If You Need Oxygen Therapy, You Can't Live a Normal Life: Many people on oxygen therapy lead active, fulfilling lives. While it may require some adjustments, portable oxygen concentrators and other advancements have made it easier for individuals to maintain mobility and independence.

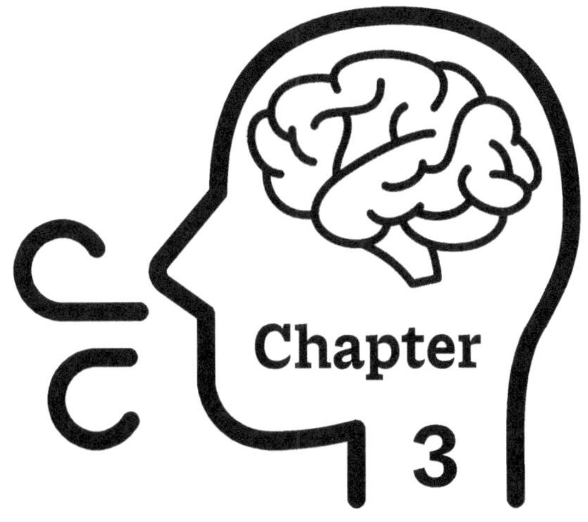

RESPIRATORY HEALTH IN SENIORS

With a relaxed breath, let your mind wander to a peaceful bamboo sanctuary, where the gentle ripple of water and the soothing chorus of birds instill a sense of serenity, guiding you into a mindful space, prepared to absorb the life-affirming lessons of breath and awareness in this chapter.

In Chapter 3, we turn our focus specifically to respiratory health in seniors, an aspect of health that is pivotal yet often overlooked. As we age, the respiratory system undergoes various changes, making the maintenance of its health increasingly important.

Understanding Respiratory Health: The importance of respiratory health cannot be overstated, especially for seniors. The lungs are our body's essential organ for oxygen exchange and keeping them healthy is crucial for maintaining quality of life. As we advance in age, our lungs and respiratory muscles gradually lose their strength and elasticity. This natural aging process can lead to decreased lung function, making it more challenging to breathe deeply and effectively. Consequently, seniors are more susceptible to respiratory infections and diseases, which can significantly impact their overall health and well-being.

Maintaining good respiratory health in the senior years involves more than just avoiding illness. It encompasses taking proactive steps to ensure that the lungs function as efficiently as possible. This includes engaging in activities and exercises that specifically target and strengthen the respiratory system.

The primary goal of this chapter is to educate readers about common respiratory issues that seniors face and provide practical, actionable strategies to address these challenges. We will delve into various conditions that can affect senior respiratory health, such as COPD, asthma, and age-related decrease in lung capacity. More importantly, we will explore how specific breathing exercises can be a powerful tool in not only managing these conditions but also in preventing some of the common respiratory problems that come with aging.

By understanding the changes that occur in the respiratory system with age and learning how to effectively counteract these changes, seniors can significantly improve their lung health. This chapter aims to empower seniors with knowledge and practical exercises to help them breathe easier, live healthier, and maintain an active lifestyle.

Age-Related Changes in the Respiratory System

As part of the normal aging process, several changes occur in the respiratory system that can affect lung capacity, muscle strength, and chest wall flexibility. Understanding these changes is vital for seniors to manage and adapt their lifestyle and healthcare routines accordingly.

Normal Aging Process: With age, the respiratory system undergoes various transformations. One of the most noticeable changes is a decrease in lung capacity. The lungs' ability to expand and contract efficiently diminishes over time, primarily due to the stiffening of the chest wall and the weakening of the respiratory muscles, including the diaphragm. Additionally, the alveoli – tiny air sacs where oxygen and carbon dioxide are exchanged – lose some of their elasticity, reducing the lungs' effectiveness in gas exchange.

Another significant change is the decline in muscle strength, including the muscles used for breathing. This decrease in muscle strength can lead to reduced stamina and endurance, making physical activities more challenging. The flexibility of the chest wall and spine also decreases, which further restricts lung expansion and reduces overall lung volume.

Impact on Breathing: These age-related changes in the respiratory system can significantly impact breathing and oxygenation in seniors. Reduced lung capacity and less efficient gas exchange mean that less oxygen is available for the body's use. This can lead to feelings of shortness of breath, particularly during physical exertion. It also means that the body must work harder to get the oxygen it needs, which can lead to increased fatigue and reduced overall energy levels.

Moreover, these changes can make seniors more susceptible to respiratory infections and conditions like chronic obstructive pulmonary disease (COPD) and pneumonia. Reduced lung function can also exacerbate other age-related health issues, such as heart disease.

Understanding these changes is crucial for seniors to take appropriate steps, such as engaging in targeted breathing exercises and leading a lung-healthy lifestyle, to mitigate the impact of these natural alterations in the respiratory system.

Common Respiratory Conditions in Seniors

As we age, our risk of developing respiratory conditions increases. Understanding these conditions is crucial for effective management and treatment. Among seniors, several respiratory issues are more prevalent, including Chronic Obstructive Pulmonary Disease (COPD), asthma, pneumonia, and sleep apnea.

Chronic Obstructive Pulmonary Disease (COPD): COPD is a common respiratory condition among seniors, characterized by persistent respiratory symptoms and airflow limitation due to airway and/or alveolar abnormalities. It usually results from significant exposure to noxious particles or gases, with smoking being the most common cause. Symptoms include shortness of breath, chronic cough, increased mucus production, and frequent respiratory infections. COPD is progressive, meaning it worsens over time, and it can significantly impact the quality of life in seniors, leading to reduced mobility and increased dependency.

Asthma in Seniors: Asthma in seniors can be a continuation of childhood asthma or newly onset asthma. It often presents differently than in younger individuals, with symptoms being less obvious and often mistaken for other age-related health issues. Seniors with asthma might experience a chronic cough, mild wheezing, or breathlessness, often leading to a delay in diagnosis and treatment. The management of asthma in seniors requires special consideration due to the presence of coexisting medical conditions and the potential for side effects from asthma medications.

Other Respiratory Issues: Pneumonia, an infection that inflames the air sacs in one or both lungs, is more common and can be more severe in seniors. Age-related changes in the immune system and lung structure increase the risk of developing pneumonia. Sleep apnea, characterized by repeated stops and starts in breathing during sleep, is another condition that can exacerbate other health issues in seniors, including heart disease and diabetes.

These conditions highlight the importance of regular health checkups, early diagnosis, and appropriate management strategies, including medication, lifestyle changes, and in some cases, breathing exercises to alleviate symptoms and improve quality of life.

The Role of Breathing Exercises in Managing Respiratory Issues

Breathing exercises play a crucial role in managing and alleviating symptoms of various respiratory conditions, especially in seniors. These exercises are designed to improve lung function, enhance airway clearance, and reduce the work of breathing. For conditions like COPD and asthma, they can be particularly beneficial.

Breathing Techniques for COPD: For individuals with COPD, exercises like pursed-lip breathing and diaphragmatic breathing are especially effective. Pursed-lip breathing involves inhaling slowly through the nose and exhaling through pursed lips, which can help slow down the breathing rate and make each breath more efficient. Diaphragmatic breathing, on the other hand, focuses on strengthening the diaphragm, the primary muscle used in breathing. This is done by breathing deeply into the lungs while consciously engaging and relaxing the diaphragm, which can help increase lung capacity and reduce the effort required to breathe.

Exercises for Asthma Relief: Gentle breathing exercises are also beneficial for managing asthma. Techniques like the Buteyko method, which involves shallow, controlled breathing, and the Papworth method, a diaphragmatic and nasal breathing technique, can help in controlling asthma symptoms. These methods focus on reducing hyperventilation, a common issue in asthma patients, thus helping to manage breathlessness and improve overall breathing efficiency.

General Exercises for Lung Health: For general lung health, exercises like deep belly breathing, rib stretch breathing, and coordinated breathing can be beneficial for various respiratory conditions. Deep belly breathing helps in fully engaging the lungs, while rib stretch breathing focuses on expanding the ribcage and improving lung capacity. Coordinated breathing, involving deep inhalation during rest and exhalation during effort, can be particularly useful for individuals engaging in physical activity.

Incorporating these exercises into a daily routine can significantly help in managing respiratory conditions, improving the quality of life for seniors with respiratory issues. It's important, however, for individuals to consult with their healthcare provider before starting any new exercise regimen, especially if they have a pre-existing respiratory condition.

Preventative Measures for Respiratory Health

Maintaining respiratory health is especially crucial for seniors, given the natural decline in lung function with age. Preventative measures play a key role in ensuring lung health and reducing the risk of respiratory conditions. Adopting certain lifestyle choices can significantly impact one's respiratory well-being.

Importance of Prevention: Preventive measures in respiratory health are vital for minimizing the risk of developing chronic conditions, managing existing issues, and enhancing overall lung function. Early prevention can lead to better health outcomes, increased longevity, and improved quality of life. For seniors, these preventative strategies are not just about avoiding illness but also about maintaining independence and the ability to engage in daily activities without respiratory limitations.

Lifestyle Choices

Smoking Cessation: Smoking is one of the most detrimental habits for lung health. It's never too late to quit smoking, as doing so can halt and even reverse some of the damage caused to the lungs. Quitting smoking reduces the risk of developing COPD, lung cancer, and other respiratory illnesses. It also improves lung function and overall health, making it one of the most important steps in respiratory health care.

Pollution Avoidance: Environmental factors play a significant role in respiratory health. Seniors should minimize exposure to pollutants, such as outdoor air pollution, secondhand smoke, and indoor pollutants like mold and dust. Using air purifiers and ensuring good ventilation can help reduce exposure to indoor pollutants.

Vaccination: Vaccinations are crucial for preventing respiratory infections, particularly in seniors. Influenza and pneumococcal vaccines are recommended as they can prevent severe lung infections and complications. Staying up to date with vaccinations is a simple yet effective way to maintain respiratory health.

In conclusion, preventive measures in respiratory health encompass a range of lifestyle choices, from quitting smoking to avoiding pollutants and staying vaccinated. By adopting these practices, seniors can significantly improve their lung health and reduce the risk of respiratory diseases.

Enhancing Lung Capacity and Strength

Improving lung capacity and strengthening the respiratory muscles are vital for seniors to maintain optimal respiratory health. Regularly performing specific exercises can significantly enhance lung function, making everyday activities easier and reducing the risk of respiratory complications.

Exercises for Improved Lung Function

Diaphragmatic Breathing: This involves focusing on and strengthening the diaphragm, the primary breathing muscle. Lie down or sit comfortably, place one hand on your belly and the other on your chest. Breathe in deeply through the nose, ensuring that the diaphragm (not the chest) expands. Exhale slowly and repeat the process.

Rib Stretch: Stand upright and breathe in deeply until you can't take in any more air. Hold for 20 seconds if possible, and then slowly exhale. This exercise allows the lungs to expand to their full capacity, stretching the muscles in your rib cage.

Blow Balloons: Blowing balloons works the abdominal and chest muscles, increasing lung capacity. It forces the lungs to work harder, thereby strengthening them.

Practical Tips

Consistency is Key: Incorporate these exercises into your daily routine for the best results. Consistency will help improve lung function over time.

Start Slowly: Begin with short sessions, gradually increasing the duration as your endurance improves.

Use Visual Aids: Visualize your lungs expanding and contracting as you breathe. This can help ensure you're doing the exercises correctly.

Stay Relaxed: Keep your body relaxed while doing these exercises. Tension, especially in the upper body, can hinder proper breathing.

Combine with Activities: Integrate breathing exercises into other daily activities, such as walking or light stretching, to make the routine more engaging and effective.

By regularly practicing these exercises and incorporating them into your daily routine, you can significantly enhance lung capacity and the strength of your respiratory muscles. This proactive approach is key to maintaining respiratory health and overall well-being in senior years.

Addressing Anxiety and Breathing Issues

The interplay between breathing and psychological states such as stress and anxiety are intricate and significant, especially as these emotional states can exacerbate respiratory issues. Understanding this relationship is crucial for managing both mental and respiratory health.

Breathing and Stress: Stress and anxiety can have a profound impact on breathing. When an individual is anxious or stressed, the body's natural response is to increase the breathing rate. This rapid, shallow breathing, often known as hyperventilation, can lead to a decrease in carbon dioxide levels in the blood, causing symptoms such as dizziness, a feeling of breathlessness, and sometimes even panic attacks. For those with existing respiratory issues, such as asthma or COPD, stress can worsen symptoms, making breathing more difficult and potentially leading to further anxiety, creating a cycle that can be challenging to break.

Relaxation Techniques: Integrating relaxation techniques into daily routines can be highly effective in managing stress-related breathing problems. Some beneficial breathing exercises include:

Diaphragmatic Breathing: By encouraging full oxygen exchange, this technique reduces the rapid, shallow breathing that often accompanies anxiety, promoting relaxation.

4-7-8 Breathing Technique: Inhale quietly through the nose for 4 seconds, hold the breath for 7 seconds, and exhale through the mouth for 8 seconds. This technique helps regulate breathing and calm the nervous system.

Progressive Relaxation: Combine deep breathing with progressively relaxing each muscle group. This can not only improve breathing patterns but also aid in overall body relaxation.

Regular practice of these techniques can help in managing stress and anxiety levels, thereby reducing their impact on breathing. It's important for individuals to find a quiet, comfortable space to practice these exercises, focusing on slow, steady breaths to maximize the benefits. By incorporating these techniques into daily life, seniors can improve their ability to manage anxiety, enhancing both their mental and respiratory health.

Nutrition and Respiratory Health

The role of nutrition in maintaining respiratory health is often underappreciated, yet it's crucial, especially for seniors. A balanced diet enriched with specific nutrients can significantly support lung function and overall respiratory health.

Dietary Considerations: Foods rich in antioxidants, vitamins, and minerals are particularly beneficial for lung health. Antioxidants combat inflammation in the body, including the lungs, and can help reduce the risk of respiratory diseases.

Fruits and Vegetables: Foods high in vitamins C, E, and beta-carotene are excellent for lung health. Examples include oranges, berries, carrots, and leafy greens. These nutrients help protect the lungs from oxidative stress and inflammation.

Omega-3 Fatty Acids: Found in fish like salmon, mackerel, and sardines, as well as flaxseeds and walnuts, omega-3 fatty acids are known for their anti-inflammatory properties, which are beneficial for respiratory health.

Whole Grains and Fiber: Whole grains, nuts, and seeds, which are high in fiber, can also support lung function. A high-fiber diet is linked to better lung health.

Magnesium-Rich Foods: Foods like almonds, spinach, and pumpkin seeds, rich in magnesium, can help improve lung function. Magnesium plays a role in relaxing bronchial muscles and regulating breathing.

Hydration and Lung Function: Adequate hydration is equally important for lung health. Water plays a crucial role in maintaining the mucosal lining in the lungs and airways. Proper hydration helps ensure that this lining stays thin enough to facilitate gas exchange while being effective in trapping dust, allergens, and pathogens, preventing them from entering the body. Dehydration can lead to thickening of this lining, which can impair lung function and make breathing more difficult.

In summary, a diet rich in antioxidants, omega-3 fatty acids, fiber, and magnesium, along with staying well-hydrated, can significantly contribute to maintaining and enhancing respiratory health in seniors. These dietary considerations, combined with other lifestyle changes, can help ensure optimal lung function and overall respiratory wellness.

Stories from Seniors

Hearing real-life experiences from seniors who have successfully managed their respiratory issues through breathing exercises can be incredibly inspiring and motivating. These stories not only showcase the effectiveness of such practices but also provide a personal touch, demonstrating how individuals have overcome their challenges.

Martha's Journey with COPD: Martha, a 72-year-old with COPD, found relief through diaphragmatic breathing. Initially skeptical, she began practicing after her therapist's recommendation. Within weeks, she noticed a significant improvement in her breathing control, especially during her daily walks. Martha shares, "I used to get winded just walking to my mailbox. Now, I can manage longer walks around the neighborhood. It's like I've regained a part of my life that I thought was over."

John's Journey with persistent sinus congestion: John, a 64-year-old who struggled with persistent sinus congestion and restricted breathing, especially at night in bed, disturbing his sleep, discovered the transformative power of alternative nostril breathing and the 4-7-8 Breathing method. Frustrated by his sinus issues and the constant feeling of congestion, he decided to explore alternative methods for relief. After researching various breathing techniques and consulting with healthcare professionals, John came across alternative nostril breathing, a practice rooted in ancient yogic traditions. With skepticism, he began to incorporate this technique when he became congested and into his daily routine.

John shared his story, saying, "I was skeptical at first, but, when I wake up congested in the middle of the night, I practice the alternative nostril breathing. At first it doesn't seem be working, but, if I keep at it, I can eventually feel my sinuses open. And like a miracle, I can breathe again with a steady flow of breathing and go back to sleep, knowing my brain is getting the proper amount of oxygen. Now, when I wake up, I feel more alert and rested. It's incredible how something as simple as focused breathing can make such a difference in my life."

George's Battle with Asthma: George, at the age of 68, had grappled with asthma for most of his adult life. Constantly searching for effective ways to manage his symptoms, he stumbled upon the benefits of pursed-lip breathing. This straightforward yet impactful technique has since become his trusted method for symptom control. George shares, "Whenever I feel an asthma attack coming on, I use this technique. It helps calm my breathing and prevents the attack from worsening." Pursed-lip breathing has become his invaluable tool for immediate relief, offering him a sense of empowerment and control over his asthma symptoms.

Susan's Recovery from Pneumonia: After battling pneumonia at the age of 75, Susan sought to regain her strength during the recovery process. She turned to a combination of rib stretch and deep belly breathing exercises. These exercises played a pivotal role in her recuperation. And Susan's commitment to regular practice resulted in a notable acceleration of her recovery and a significant enhancement of her lung capacity. Susan shared her experience, stating, "Following pneumonia, my lungs felt weak, but these exercises made all the difference. My recovery definitely accelerated, and I felt a marked improvement in my lung capacity." Susan's journey underscores the remarkable advantages that targeted breathing exercises can provide in recovery situations, facilitating the restoration of vitality and strength.

These unique, individual stories from Martha, John, George, and Susan are just a few examples of how seniors have successfully incorporated breathing exercises into their lives to manage and improve their respiratory health. They serve as a testament to the potential benefits of these practices, providing hope and encouragement to others facing similar respiratory challenges.

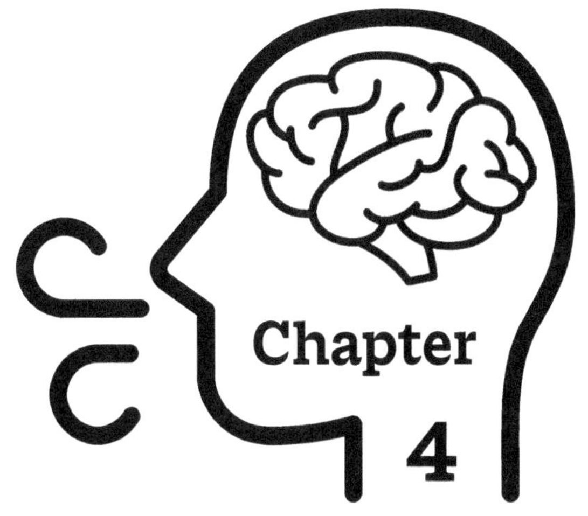

FOUNDATIONS OF BREATHING EXERCISES

With a relaxed breath, let your mind wander to a peaceful bamboo sanctuary, where the gentle ripple of water and the soothing chorus of birds instill a sense of serenity, guiding you into a mindful space, prepared to absorb the life-affirming lessons of breath and awareness in this chapter.

The primary goal of this chapter is to provide readers with a solid foundation in various breathing techniques. These will include exercises such as diaphragmatic breathing, pursed-lip breathing, and rhythmic breathing, each carefully selected for its relevance and benefit to seniors. Alongside teaching these techniques, the chapter will highlight their specific benefits, helping seniors understand how and why these exercises can improve their health.

Through a step-by-step approach, this chapter aims to equip seniors with the skills to perform these exercises effectively, making them a valuable part of their daily routine. The ultimate objective is for readers to feel confident and empowered in using these techniques to enhance their respiratory function and overall health.

Understanding Breathing Exercises

In understanding the essence and impact of breathing exercises, it's essential to recognize their purpose and the specific benefits they offer, particularly to seniors. These exercises are more than a mere routine; they are a pathway to enhanced health and well-being.

What Are Breathing Exercises: Breathing exercises involve consciously controlling the inhalation and exhalation processes in a structured manner. Unlike the automatic act of breathing, these exercises require focus and technique, aiming to improve the efficiency and effectiveness of the respiratory system. The purpose of breathing exercises is multifaceted - they are designed to strengthen the respiratory muscles, increase lung capacity, improve the efficiency of oxygen exchange, and promote relaxation of both the mind and body. These exercises can range from simple techniques like deep belly breathing to more structured practices found in yoga, such as pranayama.

Benefits for Seniors: For seniors, the benefits of breathing exercises are particularly significant.

Firstly, they help in improving lung function. As lung capacity naturally declines with age, these exercises can help mitigate this reduction, enhancing the ability to breathe deeply and fully. This improvement in lung function is crucial for maintaining energy levels and ensuring adequate oxygenation of the body.

Additionally, breathing exercises are proven to reduce stress. They activate the parasympathetic nervous system, which induces a state of relaxation, helping to lower stress and anxiety levels. This relaxation response can be particularly beneficial for seniors, contributing to improved mental health and emotional well-being.

Another key benefit is the improvement in sleep quality. The calming effect of breathing exercises can aid in reducing sleep disturbances, which are common among older adults, thereby promoting more restful and restorative sleep.

In summary, breathing exercises serve as a powerful tool for seniors, offering improved respiratory health, reduced stress levels, and better sleep quality, all of which contribute to an enhanced quality of life in the senior years.

Getting Started with Breathing Exercises

Embarking on a journey with breathing exercises requires more than just understanding their benefits; it begins with setting the right environment and approach. Proper preparation and mindfulness are key elements in maximizing the benefits of these practices, especially for seniors.

Preparation for Breathing Exercises: The first step in preparing for breathing exercises is finding a comfortable position and setting. Choose a quiet, peaceful space where you won't be disturbed. It's important that the environment feels relaxing and conducive to focus and relaxation. For the position, you can sit in a comfortable chair with your feet flat on the ground, lie down on a flat surface, or even sit cross-legged on the floor, depending on what feels best for your body. Ensure that your back is straight but not tense, and your hands rest gently in your lap or by your sides.

Next, pay attention to your clothing: Wear comfortable, loose-fitting clothes that don't restrict your breathing. If you're indoors, make sure the room has fresh air circulation, or if you're outside, find a spot with clean, fresh air, away from pollution or strong winds.

Mindfulness and Breathing: Mindfulness plays a crucial role in breathing exercises. It involves being fully present and engaged in the moment, focusing on the rhythm and depth of your breath. This concentration helps in eliminating distractions and allows you to connect more deeply with the exercise. Mindfulness enhances the relaxation benefits of the breathing exercises and ensures that you're performing them correctly, which is vital for reaping the full respiratory benefits.

Being mindful during breathing exercises also means listening to your body. If a particular technique causes discomfort, adjust your approach, or try a different exercise. Remember, the goal is to find harmony and comfort in your breathing, which in turn promotes overall health and well-being.

Starting with these foundational steps, you can effectively embark on your breathing exercise routine, ensuring a comfortable and mindful approach to each session.

Basic Breathing Techniques

For seniors looking to improve their respiratory health, mastering basic breathing techniques is a great starting point. These techniques are simple yet highly effective in enhancing lung function and overall well-being.

Diaphragmatic Breathing: Diaphragmatic breathing, or belly breathing, focuses on engaging the diaphragm actively during breathing. To practice, lie on your back with knees slightly bent, or sit comfortably in a chair. Place one hand on your belly and the other on your chest. Inhale slowly through your nose, directing the air downwards so your belly rises more than your chest. This encourages the diaphragm to do more work in aiding lung expansion. Gently exhale through pursed lips, feeling the belly fall. This technique helps deepen each breath, increase oxygen intake, and strengthen the diaphragm.

Pursed-Lip Breathing: Pursed-lip breathing is particularly helpful in controlling shortness of breath and can be used during activities that cause breathlessness. Inhale slowly through the nose for two counts, then pucker your lips as if you're going to whistle, and exhale slowly and gently through your pursed lips for a count of four or more. This technique creates a slight resistance to air flow, keeping the airways open longer and thereby improving the efficiency of each breath.

Coordinated Breathing: Coordinated breathing is especially beneficial during exercise or physical exertion. Inhale through your nose before starting an activity, and exhale through your mouth during the most strenuous part of the activity. For example, breathe in before lifting and breathe out while lifting. This coordination helps prevent holding your breath - a common issue during exertion - and maintains a steady flow of oxygen during the activity.

These basic breathing techniques are cornerstones in improving respiratory health for seniors. Regular practice can lead to noticeable improvements in breath control, lung capacity, and overall respiratory function. They can be easily integrated into daily routines, providing a simple yet effective way to boost respiratory wellness.

Building a Routine

Establishing a daily routine for breathing exercises is crucial for seniors to gain the maximum benefits. Regular practice leads to improved lung function, enhanced oxygenation, and overall well-being.

Daily Practice: The key to effective breathing exercises lies in their regularity. Integrating these exercises into your daily routine can help ensure that they become a habitual part of your day. Start by setting aside a specific time each day for practice, such as in the morning to energize and set a positive tone for the day, or in the evening to relax and improve sleep quality. Aim for at least 10-15 minutes per session.

Initially, it might be helpful to associate your breathing exercises with another daily habit, such as after brushing your teeth or before your morning coffee. This can help in forming the habit more quickly. Choose a comfortable and quiet spot where you are unlikely to be disturbed and use this same space for your exercises each day to create a sense of routine.

Tracking Progress: Keeping track of your progress can be highly motivating and can encourage consistency. Consider maintaining a breathing exercise journal where you log your daily practice, note any improvements in your breathing, and reflect on how you feel before and after each session. Over time, you might notice changes such as reduced shortness of breath during activities, improved stamina, or a greater sense of calm.

Another way to track progress is through goal setting. Set small, achievable goals at the beginning, like increasing the duration of your exercises or practicing a new technique. As you reach these goals, acknowledge your achievements, and set new ones, gradually building on your success.

Building a routine around breathing exercises and tracking your progress are instrumental in making these practices a regular and beneficial part of your life. Regular practice not only improves respiratory health but also enhances overall physical and mental well-being, making it a valuable investment in your health.

Overcoming Common Challenges

Starting breathing exercises can present challenges, especially for seniors who may already have respiratory issues or other health concerns. Understanding and addressing these challenges is key to a successful and beneficial practice.

Addressing Difficulty in Breathing: One common issue is having trouble in breathing when first starting these exercises. This can be due to various factors like pre-existing lung conditions, weakened respiratory muscles, or simply the unfamiliarity with the exercises. To overcome this, begin with very gentle, shallow breathing exercises. Focus on slow, controlled breaths rather than deep ones, gradually increasing depth as your comfort improves.

If breathlessness occurs, pause, and return to your normal breathing pattern until you feel comfortable to resume. It's important not to force or rush the process. Also, practicing in a seated position can sometimes be easier than lying down, as gravity helps the movement of the diaphragm and lungs.

Adapting Exercises to Individual Needs: When dealing with specific health conditions, it's crucial to adapt breathing exercises to meet individual needs. For instance, individuals with COPD may find pursed lip breathing particularly beneficial, while those with asthma might benefit from more relaxed, slow breathing techniques to prevent hyperventilation.

If you have a health condition that affects your breathing, consult with a healthcare professional for advice on which exercises are most suitable and safe for you. They can provide guidance on how to modify exercises to accommodate your health status and limitations. For example, people with back pain or posture issues might need to adjust their sitting or lying positions for comfort during exercises.

Remember, the goal of these exercises is not to achieve perfection but to enhance your respiratory health as much as possible within your own limits. Listening to your body and respecting its limits is crucial. With time and regular practice, you'll likely find that your capacity for these exercises grows, along with your respiratory health.

Breathing Exercises for Specific Conditions

Breathing exercises can be particularly beneficial for managing specific respiratory conditions like COPD and asthma. Tailoring these exercises to suit individual conditions can enhance their effectiveness, providing significant relief and improved quality of life for seniors.

For COPD: Seniors with Chronic Obstructive Pulmonary Disease (COPD) can benefit greatly from specific breathing exercises designed to ease breathing and improve lung function.

Pursed-Lip Breathing: This technique helps slow down the pace of breathing, making each breath more effective. Inhale slowly through the nose for two counts, then exhale through pursed lips for four counts. This creates back pressure in the airways, keeping them open longer and allowing for better air exchange.

Diaphragmatic Breathing: This focuses on strengthening the diaphragm. While sitting or lying down, place one hand on your abdomen and the other on your chest. Inhale deeply through the nose, allowing the abdomen to rise more than the chest. Exhale slowly, using the abdominal muscles to push air out of the lungs.

For Asthma: For asthma sufferers, breathing exercises can help manage symptoms and reduce the frequency of asthma attacks.

Buteyko Breathing Method: This technique involves shallow, controlled breathing to help manage breathlessness. It trains the body to breathe more slowly and deeply, reducing the tendency to hyperventilate.

Nasal Breathing: Breathing through the nose rather than the mouth can help filter out allergens and irritants. It also warms and humidifies the air, which can reduce asthma symptoms.

Relaxation and Stress-Reduction Techniques: Since stress can trigger asthma symptoms, practices like guided imagery and progressive muscle relaxation, combined with deep breathing, can be beneficial.

It's important for seniors with COPD or asthma to consult with a healthcare provider before starting any new breathing exercises, especially if their condition is severe. These exercises should be seen as complementary to, not a replacement for, prescribed medical treatments. Regular practice, under proper guidance, can significantly aid in managing these conditions and enhancing overall respiratory health.

Enhancing Exercises with Additional Techniques

Enhancing breathing exercises with additional techniques such as imagery and visualization, and incorporating gentle movements, can significantly boost their effectiveness. These techniques not only aid in relaxation but also make the exercises more engaging and beneficial.

Using Imagery and Visualization: Imagery and visualization are powerful tools that can be used to deepen the relaxation effects of breathing exercises. When practicing, seniors can imagine a serene scene, like a tranquil beach or a quiet forest.

As they breathe in, they can visualize drawing in calmness and peace from the environment, and as they breathe out, they can picture releasing stress and tension.

Another effective visualization technique involves imagining the breath as a specific color or light. For example, as you inhale, imagine a warm, soothing light filling your lungs, and as you exhale, visualize any discomfort or anxiety being expelled with the breath. This practice not only aids in relaxation but also helps maintain focus and deepens the connection with the breathing process.

Gentle Movements: Incorporating gentle movements with breathing exercises can enhance lung capacity and improve overall respiratory efficiency. Simple movements like arm raises can be synchronized with breathing: inhaling while slowly lifting the arms above the head and exhaling while lowering them. This combination helps open the chest, facilitating deeper breathing.

Another gentle movement is the seated twist, where one inhales in a neutral position and then exhales while gently twisting to one side from the waist, aiding in lung expansion and flexibility. Repeating on the other side ensures balance in the exercise.

These additional techniques not only enhance the physical benefits of breathing exercises but also bring a holistic approach, involving the mind and body, which can be particularly beneficial for seniors. By engaging both mentally and physically with the exercises, seniors can enjoy a more comprehensive and fulfilling practice.

Safety Tips and Precautions

While breathing exercises are generally safe and beneficial, there are circumstances where seniors should exercise caution. It's important to be aware of these situations and to always consult healthcare providers before starting any new exercise routine, particularly if there are pre-existing health conditions.

When to Exercise Caution: Seniors should be particularly cautious with breathing exercises during flare-ups of respiratory conditions like asthma or COPD. During these times, certain exercises might exacerbate symptoms or cause discomfort. For example, deep breathing exercises may not be suitable during an asthma attack or a severe COPD exacerbation, where it can be difficult to take deep breaths. Instead, focus on gentle, shallow breathing until the flare-up subsides.

Additionally, if you experience any dizziness, pain, or unusual shortness of breath while doing breathing exercises, it's advisable to stop immediately. These symptoms can indicate that the exercise is being performed incorrectly or that it's not suitable for your current health condition.

Consulting Healthcare Providers: Before starting a new routine of breathing exercises, it's crucial to consult with a healthcare provider, especially for seniors with underlying health conditions. A healthcare provider can offer personalized advice based on your specific health needs and limitations. They can also recommend specific exercises that would be most beneficial and safe for your condition.

It's also important to have regular check-ups with your healthcare provider to monitor your condition and to discuss the progress and effectiveness of the breathing exercises. This ongoing dialogue ensures that your exercise routine remains aligned with your health needs and goals.

Remember, while breathing exercises are a powerful tool for enhancing respiratory health, they should be practiced safely and mindfully, taking into consideration your unique health circumstances and under the guidance of a healthcare professional.

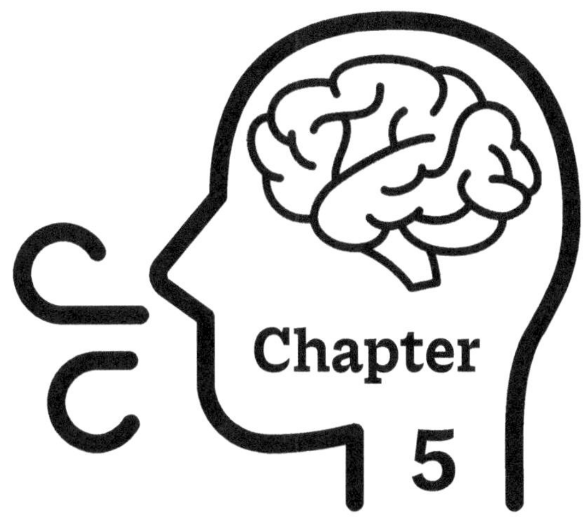

RHYTHMIC AND ENERGIZING BREATHING PRACTICES

With a relaxed breath, let your mind wander to a peaceful bamboo sanctuary, where the gentle ripple of water and the soothing chorus of birds instill a sense of serenity, guiding you into a mindful space, prepared to absorb the life-affirming lessons of breath and awareness in this chapter.

In this chapter, we delve into the invigorating world of rhythmic and energizing breathing practices. These techniques are not only vital for relaxation but also hold the power to elevate your energy levels and infuse a sense of vitality into your daily life. As seniors, maintaining a balance between relaxation and energy is essential for overall well-being.

The Power of Rhythm and Energy: Breathing is not merely an automatic bodily function; it is a potent tool that can be harnessed to influence our physical and mental states. Rhythmic and energizing breathing techniques provide us with the means to tap into this incredible power. By understanding and practicing these techniques, you can unlock new levels of relaxation, vitality, and resilience.

The rhythm of your breath has a profound impact on your body and mind. It can either calm the nervous system, promoting tranquility and rest, or awaken your senses, infusing you with renewed vigor and enthusiasm. The ability to modulate your breath in this manner gives you a remarkable degree of control over your own well-being.

Goals of the Chapter: In this chapter, our aim is twofold. Firstly, we will explore specific rhythmic breathing exercises that induce a state of profound relaxation, perfect for unwinding after a long day or promoting restful sleep. Secondly, we will delve into energizing breathing techniques designed to invigorate your body and mind, providing a natural and sustainable source of energy throughout the day.

Whether you seek the calming embrace of relaxation or the dynamic charge of energy, the exercises in this chapter offer you the means to achieve your desired state. By mastering these techniques, you will have a versatile toolkit at your disposal, ready to be employed whenever the need arises. So, let us embark on this journey of rhythmic and energizing breath, unlocking the full potential of your respiratory health and vitality.

Understanding Rhythmic Breathing

Basics of Rhythmic Breathing: Rhythmic breathing, also known as paced breathing or coherent breathing, is a breathing technique that involves consciously controlling the rhythm, depth, and pace of your breaths. It focuses on establishing a regular, even pattern of inhalation and exhalation, typically at a specific count per minute. This deliberate control over the breath serves to synchronize the body's various systems and promote a state of harmony and balance.

The fundamental principle behind rhythmic breathing is that our breath is intimately connected to our autonomic nervous system. By regulating the breath, we can influence the autonomic nervous system's response to stress. When we breathe in a steady and rhythmic manner, it signals to the body that there is no immediate threat, leading to a shift from the "fight or flight" sympathetic response to the "rest and digest" parasympathetic response. This transition promotes relaxation, reduces stress hormones, and has a calming effect on the mind and body.

BENEFITS FOR SENIORS

For seniors, rhythmic breathing offers a range of specific benefits, making it a valuable practice for managing the physical and emotional challenges that can come with aging.

These benefits include:

Improved Heart Rate Variability: Rhythmic breathing has been shown to enhance heart rate variability (HRV) in seniors. HRV is an indicator of the heart's ability to adapt to changing circumstances and is associated with better cardiovascular health and overall resilience.

Reduced Anxiety: Seniors often face increased stress and anxiety, which can negatively impact their well-being. Rhythmic breathing provides a powerful tool for reducing anxiety and promoting a sense of calm, making it easier to navigate the challenges of daily life.

By incorporating rhythmic breathing into their routines, seniors can experience not only physical benefits but also emotional well-being. This practice empowers them to manage stress, improve heart health, and enhance their overall quality of life.

Techniques for Rhythmic Breathing

Rhythmic breathing encompasses various techniques, each with its own unique benefits. In this section, we'll explore two effective rhythmic breathing techniques that can be particularly beneficial for seniors:

4-7-8 Breathing Technique: The 4-7-8 breathing technique is a simple, yet powerful method designed to promote relaxation and calmness. It's based on a specific counting pattern that regulates the breath and activates the body's relaxation response.

Here's how to practice it:

- Find a comfortable sitting or lying position.
- Close your eyes and take a deep breath in through your nose for a count of 4 seconds.
- Hold your breath for a count of 7 seconds.
- Exhale slowly and completely through your mouth for a count of 8 seconds.
- Repeat this cycle for several rounds, gradually increasing the duration as you become more comfortable with the technique.

The 4-7-8 technique is particularly effective for reducing anxiety and stress. It helps slow down racing thoughts, calm the nervous system, and induce a sense of tranquility. Seniors can use this technique whenever they feel overwhelmed or simply to unwind before bedtime.

Box Breathing: Box breathing is a method used for stress management, especially beneficial in managing anxiety and improving focus. It gets its name from the equal duration of each phase, forming a square or "box" pattern.

Here's how to practice it:

- Sit or stand comfortably with your back straight.
- Inhale through your nose for a count of 4 seconds, imagining you're tracing the first side of the box.
- Hold your breath for 4 seconds, as if you're tracing the second side.
- Exhale slowly and completely through your mouth for 4 seconds, tracing the third side.
- Pause for 4 seconds at the end of your exhale before starting the next cycle.

Box breathing brings a sense of balance and stability to the mind and body. It can be a valuable tool for seniors dealing with anxiety, as it provides a structured way to regain composure and clarity during stressful moments.

Both the 4-7-8 and box breathing techniques are easily adaptable to individual preferences and can be practiced virtually anywhere. Seniors can choose the technique that resonates with them the most and incorporate it into their daily routine to experience the soothing benefits of rhythmic breathing.

Energizing Breathing Exercises

In this section, we will explore two invigorating breathing exercises aimed at infusing seniors with vitality and mental clarity. It's important to note that while these exercises have roots in yoga and may use specialized terminology, they offer a variety of specific benefits:

Skull Shining Breath (Kapalbhati): Kapalbhati is a renowned yoga breathing technique that translates to "Skull Shining Breath." Despite its yoga origins, it can benefit seniors by awakening the mind and energizing the body.

Here's how to practice it, with modifications for seniors:

- Begin by sitting comfortably with your back straight and hands resting on your knees.
- Inhale deeply through your nose.
- Exhale forcefully and quickly through your nose while simultaneously contracting your abdominal muscles, envisioning short bursts of breath.
- Inhale passively without effort as your abdomen relaxes.
- Continue this rhythmic exhalation and passive inhalation for a designated number of breaths or a specific duration.

For seniors, it's essential to approach K Skull Shining Breath gently and avoid excessive force. You can start at a slower pace and gradually increase the speed as your comfort level improves. This exercise stimulates the abdominal muscles, enhances oxygenation, and provides an energizing effect.

Bellows Breath (Bhastrika): Bellows Breath is a dynamic and powerful breathing exercise known for increasing energy levels and clearing the mind. It offers seniors a natural way to boost vitality without resorting to stimulants.

Here's how to practice it:

- Sit comfortably with your back straight.
- Inhale deeply through your nose, filling your lungs completely.
- Exhale forcefully and quickly through your nose, expelling the breath with vigor.
- Immediately follow with a deep inhalation through your nose, filling your lungs again.
- Continue this rhythmic and vigorous breath cycle for a designated number of rounds or a specific duration.

Bellows Breath generates heat within the body, increases oxygen supply, and invigorates both the body and mind. Seniors seeking enhanced alertness and energy levels can benefit from this exercise. However, those with conditions like hypertension should practice Bellows Breath cautiously and consider consulting their healthcare provider if needed. By incorporating these energizing breathing exercises into their routines, seniors can tap into a natural reservoir of vitality and mental clarity, promoting a sense of rejuvenation and vigor in their daily lives.

Integrating Rhythmic and Energizing Practices

Creating a balanced routine that incorporates both rhythmic and energizing breathing practices can provide seniors with a comprehensive approach to enhancing their well-being.

Here are some key considerations for integrating these practices into a daily routine:

Creating a Balanced Routine: A well-rounded routine should include a mix of both calming rhythmic practices and invigorating energizing practices. Begin your session with rhythmic techniques like the 4-7-8 or box breathing to promote relaxation and reduce stress. These exercises are excellent choices to start your day or wind down in the evening.

Following the relaxation phase, consider incorporating energizing practices like Skull Shining Breath and/or Bellows Breath. These techniques can be especially beneficial during the mid-morning or mid-afternoon slump when you may need a natural energy boost. However, avoid these exercises close to bedtime to prevent overstimulation.

Listening to Your Body: It's essential for seniors to pay close attention to how their bodies respond to different breathing practices. Some days, you may find that you need more relaxation, while on others, an energy boost might be the priority. Tune into your body's signals and adjust your routine accordingly.

Seniors with specific health concerns should consult with their healthcare providers before incorporating new breathing exercises into their routines. It's crucial to ensure that the chosen practices are safe and appropriate for your individual needs and conditions.

Remember that consistency is key. Regular practice of these breathing exercises can lead to lasting benefits in terms of reduced stress, increased energy, and improved overall well-being. By creating a balanced routine and listening to your body, you can tailor your breathing practices to suit your daily requirements, helping you lead a healthier and more vibrant life as a senior.

Breathing for Emotional Balance

Breathing exercises play a significant role in regulating emotions and promoting emotional well-being for seniors. Here, we'll delve into how rhythmic and energizing breathing can positively impact mood and introduce techniques for emotional regulation:

Impact on Mood and Emotions: Rhythmic and energizing breathing techniques have a profound influence on mood and emotional states. When seniors engage in these practices, they activate the body's relaxation response, which helps reduce stress hormones like cortisol. This, in turn, fosters a sense of calmness, contentment, and emotional stability.

Regular practice of rhythmic breathing, such as the 4-7-8 or box breathing, can lead to improved emotional resilience. Seniors often find that these techniques enhance their ability to manage daily stressors, cope with anxiety, and navigate challenging emotions with greater ease.

Breathing Techniques for Emotional Regulation

Emotion Regulation Breath: This exercise involves deep, diaphragmatic breathing accompanied by the acknowledgment and labeling of emotions. Seniors can sit quietly, take deep breaths, and mentally say, "I am breathing in calmness" on the inhale and "I am releasing tension" on the exhale. This technique helps seniors process and release negative emotions.

Energizing Breath for Low Energy: When seniors are feeling low on energy or motivation, they can practice Bellows Breath to invigorate the mind and body. Bellows Breath's rapid and forceful breaths can stimulate the nervous system, increase alertness, and elevate mood.

Balancing Breath for Anxiety: To address anxiety, seniors can combine rhythmic and energizing practices. They can start with 4-7-8 breathing to induce calmness and then transition to Kapalbhati to energize and uplift their spirits.

Mindful Breath for Stress: Practicing mindfulness during rhythmic breathing exercises enhances their effectiveness in reducing stress. Seniors can focus their attention on the sensations of their breath, cultivating a sense of presence and emotional balance.

By incorporating these breathing techniques into their daily lives, seniors can develop emotional resilience, manage their moods, and find greater balance in their emotional well-being. Breathing exercises provide a valuable tool for navigating the ups and downs of life with grace and serenity.

Overcoming Challenges in Practice

While breathing exercises offer numerous benefits, seniors may encounter challenges when practicing these techniques. It's essential to address these common difficulties and provide solutions to ensure a positive and comfortable experience:

Common Difficulties and Solutions:

Difficulty with Breath Control: Seniors may initially struggle with breath control, especially when attempting rhythmic techniques. Solution: Start with shorter practice sessions and gradually extend the duration as breath control improves. Patience and consistency are key.

Shortness of Breath: Some seniors may experience shortness of breath, which can be discouraging. Solution: Choose exercises that focus on slow and deep breaths, such as diaphragmatic breathing. Avoid overly strenuous techniques.

Lack of Focus: Maintaining concentration during breathing exercises can be challenging. Solution: Practice mindfulness by gently guiding your attention back to your breath when distractions arise. Over time, your ability to stay focused will improve.

Discomfort: Seniors with physical limitations or health issues may experience discomfort during certain positions or techniques. Solution: Modify exercises to accommodate your comfort level. For example, practice breathing exercises while sitting in a chair or lying down.

Adapting Exercises for Comfort and Safety

Consult with Healthcare Provider: Seniors with specific health conditions should consult with their healthcare providers before starting a new breathing exercise routine. This step ensures that the chosen techniques are safe and suitable for individual needs.

Modifications for Physical Limitations: If you have physical limitations, adapt exercises accordingly. For example, if you have mobility issues, practice seated or lying-down breathing exercises. Modify poses in yoga-based techniques to suit your comfort level.

Breathing Aids: Some seniors may benefit from using breathing aids such as nasal strips or devices designed to improve lung function. Consult with a healthcare professional for recommendations.

Gradual Progression: Seniors who are new to breathing exercises should progress gradually. Start with simple techniques and slowly incorporate more advanced practices as you become comfortable.

Supportive Environment: Create a quiet and comfortable space for your practice. Dim lighting, calming music, or guided meditation can enhance the experience.

By addressing these challenges and adapting exercises to individual needs, seniors can enjoy the full benefits of breathing techniques while ensuring comfort and safety in their practice. Over time, consistent effort will lead to improved respiratory health and overall well-being.

The Role of Consistency and Patience

Consistency and patience are two essential pillars of successful breathing exercise practice, especially for seniors. Understanding their significance can make a significant difference in reaping the long-term benefits of these techniques.

Building a Habit: Consistent practice is the key to unlocking the full potential of breathing exercises. Seniors should strive to build a daily or regular habit of practicing these techniques. Just as one wouldn't expect immediate physical fitness results after a single workout, the benefits of breathing exercises accumulate over time. By incorporating them into daily routines, seniors can harness the power of consistent practice to enhance their respiratory health, reduce stress, and improve overall well-being.

Being Patient with Progress: Patience is equally important in the journey of mastering breathing exercises. Seniors may not experience dramatic improvements overnight, but that doesn't diminish the value of their efforts. It's essential to be patient with the progress and recognize that each day of practice contributes to long-term well-being.

Breathing exercises can offer a wide range of benefits, including improved lung function, reduced stress, enhanced emotional balance, and increased energy levels. However, these benefits may unfold gradually. Seniors should embrace the process of learning and growing in their practice, celebrating even small victories along the way.

Over time, consistent practice becomes a self-reinforcing cycle. As seniors experience the positive effects of their efforts, it motivates them to continue practicing. This positive feedback loop leads to a deeper understanding of the techniques, greater mastery, and ultimately, a higher quality of life.

In summary, consistency and patience form the foundation of a successful breathing exercise practice. By making these qualities an integral part of their journey, seniors can empower themselves to take control of their respiratory health and overall well-being, leading to a happier and healthier life.

Advanced Tips and Techniques

For seniors who are eager to take their breathing exercise practice to the next level, there are advanced tips and techniques that can deepen their experience and amplify the benefits. Here, we explore ways to enrich the practice:

Deepening the Practice

Extended Breath Holds: As seniors become more comfortable with their breathing exercises, they can experiment with extending the duration of their breath holds during techniques like the 4-7-8 breath. This extended breath retention can enhance relaxation and concentration.

Exploring Pranayama: Pranayama, the ancient yogic practice of breath control, offers a wealth of advanced breathing techniques. Seniors can explore techniques such as alternate nostril breathing or skull shining breath for profound benefits.

Meditative Breathing: Introduce meditation into your practice by incorporating mindfulness techniques. Focus on your breath and use it as an anchor for meditation, leading to enhanced mental clarity and emotional balance.

Combining with Movement

Yoga and Tai Chi: Consider integrating breathing exercises with gentle movement practices like yoga or Tai Chi. These exercises promote flexibility, balance, and coordination while synchronizing breath with movement, fostering a deeper mind-body connection.

Walking Meditation: Combine mindful walking with rhythmic breathing. With each step, synchronize your breath, allowing the rhythm of your footsteps to guide your inhalations and exhalations. This practice enhances mindfulness and grounding.

Stretching and Breath: Incorporate deep breathing into stretching routines. As you stretch and lengthen your muscles, take slow, deep breaths to enhance the stretch and promote relaxation.

Mindful Breath in Daily Activities: Extend your practice into daily life by using mindful breath during everyday activities like cooking, gardening, or doing household chores. This transforms routine tasks into opportunities for relaxation and presence.

These advanced tips and techniques offer seniors the opportunity to delve deeper into their breathing exercise practice. Whether it's through extended breath holds, the exploration of Pranayama, or the integration of breath with movement, there are endless possibilities to enrich the practice and experience even greater physical, mental, and emotional well-being.

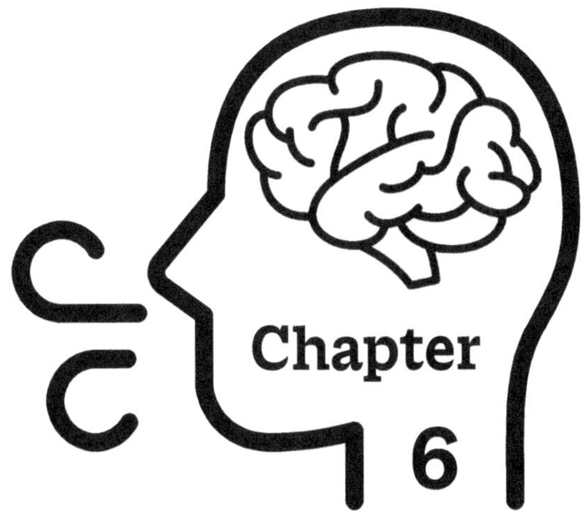

THE POWER OF YOGA BREATHING

With a relaxed breath, let your mind wander to a peaceful bamboo sanctuary, where the gentle ripple of water and the soothing chorus of birds instill a sense of serenity, guiding you into a mindful space, prepared to absorb the life-affirming lessons of breath and awareness in this chapter.

In the realm of breathing exercises, the integration of yoga and breath, known as Pranayama, holds a special place of significance. In this chapter, we will delve into the profound world of yoga breathing and its relevance for seniors. But again, please don't get turned off or hung up on the use of unfamiliar terms for yoga breathing practices. For ease of description, we will use the yoga terms in this chapter. Our aim is to equip seniors with the knowledge and practices that can bring about transformative changes in their physical, mental, and emotional well-being.

Chapter Objective: The primary objective of this chapter is to educate seniors about the immense benefits of yoga breathing and provide them with practical guidance on how to incorporate it safely into their daily lives. Yoga breathing techniques, rooted in ancient wisdom, developed, and practiced over thousands of years, offer a holistic approach to respiratory health, stress reduction, and emotional balance. As we age, these practices become even more valuable tools for maintaining vitality and a sense of inner peace.

Yoga breathing transcends the basic act of inhaling and exhaling; it's a profoundly personal journey, a connection to the very essence of our existence—the vital life force that sustains us. In the upcoming pages, you'll explore a variety of Pranayama techniques, each offering its unique personal benefits and practical applications. As a senior, you'll discover how to harness the power of your breath to increase energy, cultivate inner tranquility, and elevate your overall sense of well-being.

Safety is of utmost importance, and throughout this chapter, we will provide clear instructions and precautions to ensure that seniors can practice yoga breathing with confidence and ease. As we embark on this exploration of the breath, may seniors find not only improved respiratory health but also a deeper connection to the very essence of their being.

Understanding Breath Control (Pranayama)

What is Pranayama: Pranayama, a fundamental component of yoga, is often described as the practice of breath control. The term "Pranayama" is derived from two Sanskrit words: "Prana," which means life force or vital energy, and "Yama," which means control or regulation. Together, they signify the conscious regulation of breath to harness and direct the life force within us.

Historical and Cultural Context: Pranayama, a practice of breath control, originates from ancient India during the Vedic period (circa 1500 BCE to 500 BCE). It is mentioned in the Upanishads, some of the oldest sacred texts in both India and the world. Over time, yogic sages and scholars have refined these techniques, which continue to be practiced and evolved today.

In the cultural context of India, Pranayama is intricately connected to the concept of "Prana," which is seen as the vital life force that permeates the universe. It is believed that through Pranayama, individuals can harmonize their internal Prana, leading to physical health, mental clarity, and spiritual awakening.

Yoga, celebrated for its holistic advantages, enjoys worldwide popularity across diverse cultures. It appeals globally for enhancing physical well-being, mental calm, and personal insight. Pranayama, a central aspect of yoga focusing on breath control, is particularly noteworthy. The following chapters will specifically guide seniors through the beneficial techniques of Yoga Pranayama. These sections emphasize improvements in respiratory function, stress reduction, and spiritual growth, offering a chance to discover yoga's ancient wisdom and transformative influence.

Benefits of Yoga Breathing for Seniors

Physical and Mental Health Benefits: The practice of yoga breathing, or Pranayama, offers a multitude of benefits for seniors, encompassing both physical and mental well-being.

Improved Lung Function: Seniors often experience age-related changes in lung capacity and respiratory muscle strength. Pranayama exercises focus on expanding lung capacity and increasing oxygen intake. By practicing deep and controlled breaths, seniors can enhance their lung function, which in turn improves overall respiratory health.

Stress Reduction: Seniors face various stressors in life, from health concerns to life transitions. Yoga breathing techniques emphasize slow, deliberate breaths that activate the body's relaxation response. This leads to reduced stress levels, decreased heart rate, and a greater sense of calm and emotional stability.

Enhanced Mental Clarity: Yoga breathing enhances mental clarity and focus. The oxygenation of the brain through deep breaths promotes cognitive function, memory, and concentration. Seniors often find that regular Pranayama practice helps them stay mentally sharp and alert.

Holistic Approach to Well-being: Yoga, including the practice of Pranayama, embraces a holistic approach to well-being. It recognizes that health is not solely a physical aspect but also involves mental and spiritual dimensions. By incorporating yoga breathing into their lives, seniors can experience a comprehensive sense of vitality and balance.

Key Pranayama Techniques

In this chapter, seniors will delve into key Pranayama techniques, each offering unique benefits for their physical and mental well-being. These techniques are accessible, gentle, and tailored to the needs of seniors.

Alternate Nostril Breathing (Anulom Vilom)

To practice Alternate Nostril Breathing, seniors can follow these simple steps:

- Sit comfortably with an upright spine.

- Use the right thumb to close the right nostril and the right ring finger to close the left nostril.

- Start by inhaling deeply through both nostrils.

- Close the right nostril with the thumb and exhale slowly and completely through the left nostril.

- Inhale through the left nostril.

- Close the left nostril with the ring finger and exhale slowly through the right nostril.

- This completes one cycle. Continue for 5-10 cycles, gradually extending the duration.

    Benefits: Alternate Nostril Breathing is known for its ability to balance the left and right hemispheres of the brain, promoting mental clarity and emotional balance. It also helps in reducing stress and anxiety.

Ocean Breath (Ujjayi Breath):

How to perform: Ocean Breath is performed by gently constricting the back of the throat to create a soft, ocean-like sound during both inhalation and exhalation. It can be practiced in a seated or lying position.

Benefits: Ocean Breath is a soothing and calming technique that can help seniors achieve a sense of relaxation and presence. It is often used in yoga practices to synchronize breath with movement.

Bee Breath (Bhramari):

Practice guidelines: To practice Bee Breath, seniors can sit comfortably with their eyes closed. They gently close their ears with their thumbs, place their index fingers on their forehead, and the remaining fingers on their eyes. Taking a deep breath in, they exhale while making a humming sound like the buzzing of a bee.

Benefits: Bee Breath is an effective technique for instant stress relief and relaxation. The humming sound and the gentle vibrations it creates have a calming effect on the nervous system.

Seniors will find these Pranayama techniques not only accessible but also highly effective in promoting relaxation, mental clarity, and emotional well-being. As they explore and incorporate these techniques into their daily routines, they will discover the transformative power of yoga breathing in their lives.

Adapting Yoga Breathing for Seniors

As seniors embark on their journey into the world of Pranayama, it's essential to understand that yoga breathing can be adapted to suit their unique needs and circumstances. Here, we explore how seniors can modify and practice Pranayama safely and effectively:

Modifications and Precautions:

- Seated Position: Seniors can perform Pranayama in a comfortable seated position, either on a chair or a cushion. This eliminates the need to sit on the floor, making it more accessible.

- Gentle Movements: Incorporating gentle movements or stretches alongside Pranayama can enhance flexibility and reduce the risk of stiffness. These movements should be slow and controlled.

- Breath Duration: Seniors can start with shorter breath cycles and gradually extend them as they become more comfortable. It's essential not to push beyond their comfort zone.

- Props: Props like cushions or blankets can provide support and comfort during Pranayama practice, especially for those with mobility issues.

- Health Considerations: Seniors with specific health concerns should consult with their healthcare provider before starting any new breathing exercises. Conditions like high blood pressure or heart issues may require special precautions.

Listening to Your Body

One of the fundamental principles of practicing yoga breathing, especially for seniors, is listening to one's body. It's crucial to be attuned to how the body responds during Pranayama and adjust accordingly.

Here are some key points to keep in mind.

Discomfort vs. Challenge: Seniors should distinguish between discomfort and challenge. While some level of challenge is beneficial for growth, discomfort or pain is a sign to ease off or modify the practice.

Breathing Rate: The breath should always be smooth and controlled. If seniors find themselves gasping for air or feeling dizzy, it's essential to slow down and return to normal breathing.

Consistency: Seniors should aim for consistency in their practice. Regular but moderate practice is more beneficial than sporadic intense sessions.

Progress: Progress in yoga breathing may be slow and incremental, especially for seniors. It's crucial to remain patient and not be discouraged by perceived limitations.

By modifying Pranayama practices to accommodate age-related limitations and by listening to their bodies, seniors can safely and effectively incorporate yoga breathing into their daily routines. This adaptation ensures that Pranayama becomes a valuable tool in their journey toward improved respiratory health and overall well-being.

Integrating Pranayama into Daily Life

Pranayama, the art of yoga breathing, holds immense potential for enhancing seniors' respiratory health and overall well-being. To reap the full benefits, it's essential to integrate Pranayama into daily life effectively.

Here's how seniors can make yoga breathing a seamless part of their routines:

Start by Creating a Daily Routine

Consistent Timing: Choose a consistent time each day for Pranayama practice. Many find it beneficial to practice in the morning to start the day with a sense of calm and clarity.

Set an Intention: Before each session, set a positive intention or affirmation. This helps create a focused and purposeful practice.

Start Slowly: Begin with a few minutes of Pranayama and gradually increase the duration as comfort levels and familiarity grow.

Incorporate Triggers: Link Pranayama to daily triggers like waking up, having a cup of tea, or winding down before bedtime. These triggers serve as reminders to practice.

Combining with Meditation and Mindfulness

Mindful Breathing: Merge Pranayama with mindfulness by paying close attention to each breath. Focus on the sensation of the breath entering and leaving the body.

Meditation: Following a Pranayama session, transition into a short meditation. Meditation can deepen the sense of inner peace and stillness achieved through controlled breathing.

Body Scan: Combine Pranayama with a body scan meditation, where you systematically relax each part of the body. This enhances overall relaxation and reduces tension.

Visualization: During Pranayama, incorporate visualization techniques, such as imagining a tranquil place or envisioning the breath cleansing and rejuvenating the body.

Gratitude Practice: Conclude your practice with a moment of gratitude, reflecting on the positive aspects of your life. This promotes a sense of contentment and positivity.

By weaving Pranayama into daily routines and enhancing it with meditation and mindfulness, seniors can experience a profound transformation in their respiratory health and overall quality of life. The integration of these practices fosters not only physical well-being but also mental and emotional balance, leading to a harmonious and fulfilling daily life.

Overcoming Common Challenges

Practicing Pranayama, the art of yoga breathing, can bring about transformative benefits for seniors, but it's important to address common challenges that may arise during the journey:

Breathing Difficulties and Solutions:

Shortness of Breath: Seniors with respiratory issues may initially experience shortness of breath. Start with gentle techniques like Alternate Nostril Breathing and gradually progress to more advanced ones as comfort levels improve.

Physical Limitations: Age-related limitations or health conditions may restrict certain movements. Modify Pranayama poses as needed to ensure safety and comfort.

Fatigue: If fatigue sets in, reduce the duration of each session and practice more frequently. Consistency is more important than intensity.

Lightheadedness: Some seniors may feel lightheaded during deep breathing exercises. In such cases, practice sitting down and avoid overly forceful breaths.

Staying Motivated

Set Goals: Define clear, achievable goals for your Pranayama practice. Whether it's improving lung capacity, reducing stress, or enhancing overall well-being, having objectives keeps you motivated.

Accountability: Partner with a friend or family member who shares your interest in yoga breathing. Practicing together can provide motivation and a sense of community.

Variety: Explore different Pranayama techniques to keep your practice fresh and engaging. Variety prevents boredom and maintains enthusiasm.

Progress Tracking: Keep a journal to track your progress. Note any improvements in lung capacity, reduced stress levels, or enhanced relaxation. Celebrate small victories along the way.

Mindfulness Practice: Combine Pranayama with mindfulness exercises. The awareness cultivated through mindfulness can deepen your connection to the practice and boost motivation.

Incorporate Music or Guided Sessions: Listen to soothing music or guided Pranayama sessions to add an element of enjoyment and structure to your practice.

By addressing breathing difficulties with sensitivity and implementing strategies to stay motivated, seniors can overcome challenges and fully embrace the transformative power of Pranayama. This holistic approach to respiratory health not only enhances physical well-being but also fosters mental and emotional balance, creating a fulfilling and sustainable wellness routine.

The Role of Guidance and Community

Embarking on a journey to explore the benefits of Pranayama, or yoga breathing, can be greatly enriched by guidance and community support:

Finding a Breathing Coach or Yoga Instructor

Qualifications Matter: Look for a breathing or yoga instructor who specializes in teaching seniors. They should have the necessary certifications and experience to tailor practices to the unique needs and limitations of older adults.

Ask for Recommendations: Seek recommendations from friends, family, or healthcare professionals who may know of reputable instructors. Word-of-mouth referrals often lead to trusted instructors.

Check Credentials: Ensure that the instructor is certified by a recognized association and has a background in adapting breathing and yoga practices for seniors.

Interview Potential Instructors: Schedule introductory meetings or consultations with prospective instructors to discuss your goals, any health concerns, and their teaching approach. This allows you to gauge their compatibility with your needs.

Community and Group Practices

The Power of Group Dynamics: Participating in group breathing and yoga classes can provide a sense of belonging and motivation. Being part of a community of like-minded individuals can boost enthusiasm and commitment to the practice.

Shared Experiences: In a group setting, you can share your experiences, challenges, and progress with others. This sharing can foster a sense of solidarity and encourage continuous improvement.

Guided Practice: Group classes led by experienced instructors ensure that you receive proper guidance and alignment cues. This is especially important for seniors who may require adjustments to poses and techniques.

Social Interaction: Breathing and Yoga classes offer an opportunity for social interaction, which is beneficial for mental and emotional well-being. Building friendships within the class community can add an enjoyable social aspect to your wellness journey.

Variety of Practices: Group classes often include a variety of Yoga Breathing (Pranayama) techniques and yoga poses. This diversity keeps your practice interesting and allows you to explore different aspects of health activities like yoga.

Incorporating guidance from a qualified instructor and engaging in group practices can enhance your experience with breathing practices (Pranayama), providing you with the expertise and support needed to fully embrace the profound benefits of yoga breathing. Whether you choose individual or group sessions, both paths offer valuable opportunities for growth, connection, and holistic well-being.

Advanced Yoga Breathing (Pranayama) Techniques

For those who have developed a strong foundation in Yoga breathing techniques (Pranayama) and are looking to deepen their practice, there are advanced techniques that can offer profound benefits. However, it's crucial to approach these techniques with caution, patience, and under the guidance of an experienced instructor.

Safety and Precautions: Advanced Pranayama techniques require a solid foundation in basic Pranayama and yoga practice. It's essential to progress slowly, respect your body's limitations, and never force any technique. Always practice advanced Pranayama under the guidance of an experienced yoga instructor who can provide personalized instructions and monitor your progress. If you have any underlying health conditions, consult with your healthcare provider before attempting advanced Pranayama practices to ensure they are safe for you.

As you explore these advanced techniques, remember that Pranayama is a journey of self-discovery and inner transformation. Approach your practice with reverence, mindfulness, and a deep respect for your own body and mind.

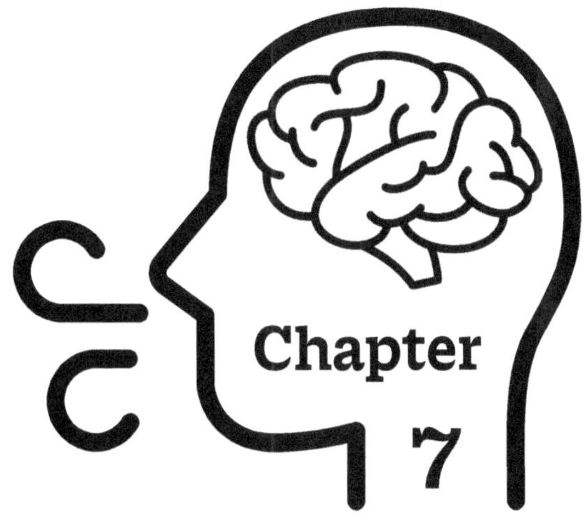

Chapter 7

INTEGRATING BREATHING INTO DAILY LIFE

With a relaxed breath, let your mind wander to a peaceful bamboo sanctuary, where the gentle ripple of water and the soothing chorus of birds instill a sense of serenity, guiding you into a mindful space, prepared to absorb the life-affirming lessons of breath and awareness in this chapter.

In the fast-paced world we live in, it's easy to overlook the simple yet profound act of breathing. However, for seniors, integrating breathing exercises into daily life can be a transformative practice that enhances well-being on multiple levels. This chapter is dedicated to highlighting the importance of daily practice and offering guidance on how seniors can seamlessly incorporate breathing exercises into their routines.

The Importance of Daily Practice: The benefits of breathing exercises extend beyond the moments spent in practice; they have the potential to positively impact every aspect of a senior's life. Daily practice not only strengthens lung function and reduces stress but also instills a sense of mindfulness that carries over into daily activities. It fosters a heightened awareness of the present moment, leading to better decision-making, increased emotional resilience, and improved overall health.

Chapter Goals: The primary goal of this chapter is to empower seniors with practical strategies for integrating breathing exercises into their daily lives. From the moment they wake up to the moment they rest, seniors will discover how to infuse each day with mindful breath. Whether it's the gentle art of mindful breathing while sipping morning tea, the rejuvenating power of midday breathing breaks, or the tranquility of evening relaxation exercises, this chapter will provide a comprehensive guide to making breath a constant companion.

As we embark on this journey of seamlessly integrating the wisdom of breath into daily life, seniors will find that the ordinary becomes extraordinary, the mundane becomes sacred, and each breath becomes a source of vitality, clarity, and inner peace.

Establishing a Breathing Routine

Building a Daily Breathing Schedule: The foundation of integrating breathing exercises into daily life lies in creating a structured schedule. Seniors should aim to establish a routine that suits their lifestyle and preferences. Start by selecting specific times during the day for breathing exercises. For many, mornings are ideal for setting a positive tone for the day. Midday breaks provide an opportunity to recharge and refocus, while evening practices can promote relaxation and restful sleep.

It's crucial to choose times that align with personal habits. For example, integrating breathing exercises into existing routines, such as during morning coffee or evening reading, can make them feel like a natural part of the day. Setting alarms or reminders on a phone or placing visual cues like sticky notes can also help seniors remember to practice.

Consistency Over Intensity: One of the keys to successful integration is consistency. It's more effective to practice breathing exercises daily for a shorter duration than sporadically for extended periods. Consistency allows seniors to reap the cumulative benefits of breathing exercises, such as improved lung function, reduced stress, and enhanced overall well-being.

While intensity and duration can be gradually increased as seniors become more comfortable with the practice, it's essential to prioritize regularity over pushing oneself too hard. Short, focused sessions can be incredibly effective and manageable, even for those with busy schedules.

By establishing a breathing routine that aligns with daily life and emphasizing consistency, seniors can harness the transformative power of breath to enhance their physical and mental well-being, making it a lifelong habit for health and vitality.

Incorporating Breathing Exercises into Various Activities

During Morning Rituals: The mornings set the tone for the day, and incorporating breathing exercises into morning rituals can be an invigorating start. Seniors can begin by finding a quiet and comfortable spot to sit or stand. A few minutes of deep diaphragmatic breathing, where they inhale deeply through the nose, filling their lungs, and exhale slowly through pursed lips, can awaken their senses and provide mental clarity. This practice helps seniors transition from sleep to an alert and focused state.

While Engaging in Physical Activity: Seniors who engage in physical activities like walking, stretching, or yoga can integrate breathing exercises seamlessly. For instance, during a morning walk, they can synchronize their breath with their steps. Inhaling for a few steps and exhaling for the same number of steps helps maintain a rhythmic and energizing pace. Stretching exercises can be enhanced by pairing each stretch with a deep breath, promoting relaxation and flexibility. By syncing breath with movement, seniors can increase oxygen intake, making physical activities more efficient and enjoyable.

During Relaxation and Leisure Time: Leisure activities offer an excellent opportunity to incorporate breathing exercises. Seniors can practice gentle breathing techniques while reading a book, tending to a garden, or even watching a favorite TV show. For instance, during moments of relaxation, they can indulge in calming techniques like the 4-7-8 breathing exercise, helping them unwind and reduce stress. These practices enhance the enjoyment of leisure activities while providing significant mental and emotional benefits.

By seamlessly integrating breathing exercises into various daily activities, seniors can experience the advantages of enhanced lung function, reduced stress, and heightened mindfulness throughout their day. These techniques become valuable companions, enriching their daily routines and overall well-being.

Breathing Exercises for Different Times of the Day

Morning Energizers: Mornings can set the tone for the entire day, and starting with invigorating breathing exercises can provide seniors with a burst of energy. The "Breath of Fire" technique from yoga is an excellent choice. To practice this, seniors can sit comfortably with an upright posture, place their hands on their diaphragm, and take quick, rhythmic breaths through the nose, emphasizing exhalation. This technique oxygenates the body, increases alertness, and prepares seniors for an active day.

Afternoon Refreshers: Afternoons often bring a dip in energy levels. To combat this, seniors can practice what is called "Equal Breath". This involves inhaling and exhaling for the same count, such as inhaling for a count of four and exhaling for a count of four. This technique stabilizes the nervous system, reduces stress, and re-energizes the body. Seniors can do this seated at their desk, in a quiet corner, or even during a short break.

Evening Relaxation Practices: Evenings are a time for winding down and preparing for restful sleep. Breathing exercises can play a crucial role in achieving relaxation. The "4-7-8" technique is highly effective. Seniors can sit or lie down comfortably and inhale quietly through the nose for a count of four, hold the breath for a count of seven, and exhale slowly and audibly through the mouth for a count of eight.

This practice promotes deep relaxation, reduces anxiety, and aids in falling asleep peacefully.

By tailoring breathing exercises to different times of the day, seniors can harness the power of breath to enhance their energy levels, reduce stress, and ensure a peaceful night's sleep. These practices become valuable tools in maintaining vitality and emotional balance throughout the day.

Overcoming Barriers to Practice

Dealing with Physical Limitations: It's essential to acknowledge that not all seniors have the same physical abilities, and some may face limitations that affect their practice of breathing exercises. However, there are numerous modifications and variations that can make breathing exercises accessible to individuals with physical challenges.

For seniors with mobility issues, seated breathing exercises can be highly effective. These exercises can be done while sitting in a chair or wheelchair, ensuring comfort and stability. Additionally, seniors can use props such as pillows or bolsters to support their posture and make the practice more accessible. For those with reduced upper body strength, focusing on diaphragmatic breathing can be particularly beneficial, as it doesn't require extensive physical effort.

Addressing Lack of Motivation: Motivation can be a common barrier to consistent practice. Seniors may initially feel enthusiastic about incorporating breathing exercises into their daily routines but struggle to maintain that enthusiasm over time. To address this challenge, it's essential to emphasize the importance of setting achievable goals.

Seniors can start with small, manageable goals, such as practicing a specific breathing exercise for just a few minutes each day. Gradually, they can increase the duration and complexity of their practice as they become more comfortable and motivated. Encouraging seniors to track their progress and celebrate their achievements, no matter how small, can also boost motivation.

Furthermore, seniors can benefit from the support of a buddy or caregiver who can join them in their breathing exercises. Having someone to share the experience with can make the practice more enjoyable and provide mutual motivation.

Tracking and Measuring Progress

Journaling and Reflecting: One effective way for seniors to track and measure their progress with breathing exercises is to maintain a dedicated journal. Journaling allows individuals to document their daily practice, thoughts, and experiences related to breathing exercises. Here's how seniors can benefit from this practice:

Recording Practice Sessions: Seniors can use their journal to note the duration and type of breathing exercises they perform each day. This provides a clear record of their commitment to the practice.

Tracking Physical Sensations: Encourage seniors to describe how their body feels before and after each session. Do they notice any changes in muscle tension, posture, or breathing patterns? Documenting these physical sensations can help individuals become more aware of their bodies.

Emotional Well-being: Breathing exercises can have a profound impact on emotional well-being. Seniors can use their journal to express their feelings before and after practicing. Did they experience reduced stress, increased relaxation, or improved mood? Reflecting on these emotional changes can be enlightening.

Progress Over Time: By regularly reviewing their journal entries, seniors can observe trends and improvements in their practice. They may notice that they can perform certain exercises for longer durations, experience less breathlessness, or have better control over their breath.

Recognizing Improvements: Recognizing and celebrating improvements is a crucial aspect of sustaining motivation and commitment to breathing exercises. Seniors can follow these steps to acknowledge their progress:

Set Milestones: Encourage seniors to set achievable milestones for their practice. For example, they can aim to increase their practice duration by a minute each week or reduce stress levels by a certain percentage.

Celebrate Small Wins: Emphasize the importance of celebrating even small achievements. Whether it's successfully completing a challenging breathing exercise or feeling more relaxed after a session, each step forward is a reason to celebrate.

Seek Feedback: Seniors can ask their caregivers or loved ones for feedback on changes they've observed. External validation of their progress can boost their confidence and motivation.

Visualize Progress: Visualization techniques can help seniors imagine the positive impact of their practice on their overall well-being. Encourage them to picture themselves achieving their goals and enjoying better health.

Incorporating journaling and recognizing improvements into their breathing exercise routine can provide seniors with a sense of accomplishment and motivation to continue their practice. This self-awareness and positive reinforcement contribute to the long-term success of their respiratory health journey.

Mindfulness and Breathing

The Role of Mindfulness: Mindfulness is a state of focused awareness on the present moment, without judgment. When combined with breathing exercises, mindfulness can significantly enhance their effectiveness for seniors. Here's why mindfulness plays a crucial role:

Enhanced Presence: Mindfulness encourages seniors to be fully present during their breathing practice. Instead of letting their minds wander, they learn to anchor their attention to the sensations of breathing, promoting a deeper connection with the exercise.

Stress Reduction: Mindful breathing can be a powerful stress-reduction tool. It allows seniors to observe their thoughts and emotions without reacting to them. This awareness enables them to manage stress more effectively and make conscious choices in response to challenging situations.

Improved Concentration: For seniors concerned about cognitive function, mindfulness can enhance concentration and cognitive clarity. It sharpens their ability to focus on the breath, which can, in turn, have a positive impact on memory and cognitive function.

Mindful Breathing Techniques

Counted Breaths: Instruct seniors to count their breaths as they inhale and exhale. For example, they can silently count to four during inhalation and four during exhalation. This counting keeps their attention on the breath and away from distractions.

Body Scan: Encourage seniors to perform a body scan while breathing. Starting from their toes and moving up to the head, they should focus on each body part, noticing any tension or sensations. This practice promotes body awareness and relaxation.

Noting Thoughts: Seniors can practice noting thoughts as they arise during their breathing exercise. Instead of getting caught up in the thought, they acknowledge it and then gently return their attention to the breath. This technique helps seniors detach from racing thoughts.

Guided Meditation: Provide guided mindfulness meditation sessions specifically designed for seniors. These sessions can lead seniors through a series of mindfulness exercises, gradually deepening their practice.

By integrating mindfulness with breathing exercises, seniors can experience a holistic approach to well-being. They learn to appreciate the present moment, reduce stress, and enhance their overall quality of life through the power of mindful breathing.

Breathing Exercises for Specific Needs

Breathing exercises tailored to specific needs can be powerful tools for seniors to address stress relief and improve sleep. Here are some effective techniques for each purpose:

For Stress Relief:

Deep Abdominal Breathing (Diaphragmatic Breathing): This fundamental technique involves breathing deeply into the abdomen. Seniors can practice it by inhaling slowly through the nose for a count of four, allowing the abdomen to expand, and exhaling for a count of six, releasing tension. This exercise activates the body's relaxation response and reduces stress.

4-7-8 Breathing: Instruct seniors to breathe in for a count of four, hold the breath for a count of seven, and exhale slowly for a count of eight. This technique calms the nervous system and is effective in reducing anxiety.

Belly Breathing with Visualization: Combine diaphragmatic breathing with visualization. Seniors can imagine inhaling positivity and exhaling stress or negativity. This practice engages the mind in a positive way while promoting relaxation.

For Improved Sleep:

Box Breathing: Seniors can practice this method before bedtime. Inhale for a count of four, hold for four, exhale for four, and then pause for four before starting the cycle again. It regulates the breath and prepares the body for restful sleep.

Progressive Muscle Relaxation: While not a pure breathing exercise, it involves deep breathing alongside muscle relaxation. Seniors can tense and release different muscle groups while taking slow, deep breaths. This technique can relieve physical tension that may interfere with sleep.

Guided Imagery and Breath: Combine deep breathing with guided imagery that transports seniors to a peaceful place. Inhaling slowly while mentally picturing calming scenes can ease the mind and improve sleep quality.

These targeted breathing exercises empower seniors to manage stress and enhance sleep naturally. Encourage them to choose the technique that resonates most with their needs and integrate it into their daily routines for lasting benefits. By practicing these exercises regularly, seniors can enjoy reduced stress and improved sleep, leading to a better overall quality of life.

Integrating Breathing with Other Wellness Practices

Breathing exercises can be seamlessly integrated with other wellness practices, enhancing their overall effectiveness, and contributing to a holistic approach to health and well-being.

Here's how seniors can combine breathing exercises with meditation, yoga, and a broader holistic health plan:

Combining with Meditation or Yoga: Mindful Meditation: Seniors can start a meditation session with a few minutes of deep breathing to calm the mind and enhance focus. The rhythm of the breath serves as an anchor for meditation, making it easier to enter a meditative state.

Yoga and Pranayama: For those practicing yoga, combining yoga postures (asanas) with specific Pranayama techniques can deepen the mind-body connection. For example, pairing a relaxation-focused breath like "4-7-8" with gentle stretches or restorative yoga poses can promote relaxation and flexibility.

Breath Awareness: In both meditation and yoga, seniors can maintain continuous awareness of their breath. This practice fosters mindfulness and helps individuals stay present during their sessions.

Incorporating into a Holistic Health Plan

Diet and Nutrition: Proper nutrition plays a vital role in overall health, including lung health. Seniors can integrate breathing exercises with mindful eating practices. Deep breaths before meals can promote digestion and enhance the enjoyment of food.

Physical Activity: Regular exercise, tailored to individual needs and abilities, is essential for seniors. Breathing exercises can be incorporated into pre-exercise warm-ups and post-exercise cool-downs to optimize lung function.

Stress Management: Stress reduction is a cornerstone of holistic health. Seniors can use breathing exercises as a tool to manage stress, thereby reducing its negative impact on their physical and mental well-being.

Hydration: Adequate hydration is crucial for lung health. Seniors can practice deep breathing while sipping water to ensure they are staying hydrated throughout the day.

By combining breathing exercises with meditation, yoga, and other aspects of a holistic health plan, seniors can experience synergistic benefits. These practices work in harmony to promote physical, mental, and emotional well-being, providing a comprehensive approach to health that supports a vibrant and fulfilling life in the senior years.

Throughout this book, we have explored the science of breath, its profound impact on physical and mental health, and a rich tapestry of techniques, from deep diaphragmatic breaths to the rhythmic dances of Pranayama. We've learned how to adapt these practices to individual needs and integrate them into daily life.

Breathing exercises can:

- Improve lung function and oxygenate your body.

- Reduce stress, anxiety, and promote relaxation.

- Enhance cognitive function and emotional well-being.

- Help manage and prevent respiratory issues.

- Energize and vitalize your body.

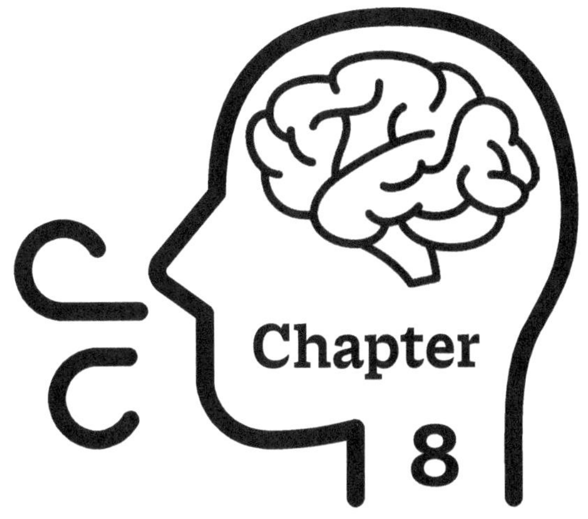

NUTRITION, HYDRATION, AND EXERCISE

With a relaxed breath, let your mind wander to a peaceful bamboo sanctuary, where the gentle ripple of water and the soothing chorus of birds instill a sense of serenity, guiding you into a mindful space, prepared to absorb the life-affirming lessons of breath and awareness in this chapter.

Holistic Approach to Respiratory Health

Breathing is the essence of life, but its efficacy is intricately tied to the body's overall health. A holistic approach acknowledges that the body functions as a unified whole. Just as breathing exercises enrich the body and mind, so too do the choices we make about what we eat, drink, and how we move.

Three Pillars to Respiratory Health:

Nutrition: We'll delve into the world of foods that nourish the lungs and support their function. From antioxidants that combat inflammation to nutrients that promote lung elasticity, we'll explore the dietary choices that can enhance your respiratory well-being.

Hydration: Water is life, and proper hydration is essential for optimal lung function. We'll discuss the significance of staying well-hydrated and how it can affect your breathing and overall health.

Exercise: Physical activity is not only about keeping your muscles strong but also about invigorating your lungs. We'll explore exercises that can improve lung capacity, enhance oxygen utilization, and keep your respiratory system in top form.

The Role of Nutrition in Respiratory Health

Importance of a Balanced Diet: A balanced diet serves as the cornerstone of good health, and its impact on respiratory well-being cannot be overstated. For seniors, maintaining a well-rounded and nutritious diet is particularly crucial. A balanced diet provides the body with the essential nutrients it needs for growth, repair, and optimal function. This balance extends to all aspects of health, including respiratory health.

As we age, our bodies undergo natural changes, including a decrease in muscle mass and a potential decline in lung function. These changes can make seniors more vulnerable to respiratory issues. However, a well-balanced diet can play a pivotal role in mitigating these effects and promoting lung health.

Nutrients Beneficial for Lung Health: Several nutrients have been identified as beneficial for lung health, and seniors should prioritize including them in their diet:

Antioxidants: Antioxidant-rich foods such as fruits and vegetables help combat oxidative stress and inflammation in the respiratory system. Berries, leafy greens, and citrus fruits are excellent choices.

Omega-3 Fatty Acids: Foods like fatty fish (salmon, mackerel) and flaxseeds contain omega-3 fatty acids, which have anti-inflammatory properties and may support lung function.

Vitamin C: This vitamin, found in abundance in citrus fruits, plays a vital role in lung health by protecting against oxidative damage and supporting the immune system.

Vitamin E: Nuts, seeds, and vegetable oils are rich in vitamin E, which can help protect lung cells from damage.

Magnesium: Magnesium-rich foods like nuts, seeds, and whole grains contribute to lung health by relaxing the airways and promoting easier breathing.

Fiber: High-fiber foods like whole grains and legumes can help maintain a healthy weight, reducing the risk of respiratory issues related to obesity.

By incorporating these nutrient-rich foods into their diets, seniors can enhance their lung health and reduce the risk of respiratory problems. In this chapter, we'll delve deeper into specific dietary recommendations and practical tips to help seniors make informed and health-conscious choices for their respiratory well-being.

Hydration and Lung Function

The Importance of Staying Hydrated: Proper hydration is not only essential for overall health but also plays a vital role in maintaining optimal lung function and supporting the respiratory system. The lungs are lined with a thin layer of mucus, which serves as a natural defense mechanism. This mucus traps and clears irritants, pathogens, and particles from the air we breathe. However, for this defense mechanism to work effectively, it requires adequate hydration.

When the body is well-hydrated, the mucus in the airways remains thin and slippery. This consistency allows the mucus to move freely and efficiently, facilitating the removal of unwanted substances from the respiratory tract. In contrast, dehydration can lead to thicker and stickier mucus, impairing its ability to perform its protective function. This can make the respiratory system more susceptible to infections and irritants.

Furthermore, staying properly hydrated helps maintain the elasticity of lung tissue. The lungs contain small air sacs called alveoli, which need to remain pliable for efficient oxygen exchange. Dehydration can cause these tissues to become stiff and less effective in oxygenating the blood.

Tips for Adequate Hydration

Ensuring seniors stay adequately hydrated is essential for their respiratory health. Here are some practical tips to help seniors maintain proper hydration:

Drink Water Regularly: Encourage seniors to sip water throughout the day, even if they don't feel thirsty. Setting reminders or using water bottles with measurements can help track daily intake.

Incorporate Hydrating Foods: Foods with high water content, such as fruits (watermelon, oranges) and vegetables (cucumbers, celery), can contribute to hydration.

Limit Dehydrating Beverages: Reduce the consumption of beverages that can contribute to dehydration, such as caffeinated and alcoholic drinks.

Monitor Urine Color: Light yellow urine is a good indicator of proper hydration. Dark yellow or amber urine may signal dehydration.

Consider Special Needs: Seniors with certain medical conditions, like diabetes or kidney disease, may have unique hydration requirements. Consultation with a healthcare provider is advisable.

By maintaining adequate hydration, seniors can support their lung health, ensure efficient mucus clearance, and optimize lung tissue elasticity, contributing to overall respiratory well-being. This chapter will delve further into the intersection of hydration, nutrition, and respiratory health, providing seniors with a comprehensive guide to holistic lung care.

Physical Exercise and Lung Health

Benefits of Regular Exercise: Regular physical exercise is a cornerstone of maintaining good lung health, especially for seniors.

Engaging in physical activity provides a wide range of benefits for the respiratory system and overall well-being:

Improved Lung Capacity: Exercise encourages deep breathing and the expansion of the lungs, which can enhance lung capacity. This means that the lungs can take in more oxygen and expel more carbon dioxide with each breath.

Enhanced Respiratory Efficiency: Physical activity increases the demand for oxygen in the body. Over time, this can lead to improved efficiency in oxygen uptake and utilization by the lungs.

Strengthening Respiratory Muscles: Exercises like walking, swimming, and yoga engage the respiratory muscles, including the diaphragm and intercostal muscles. Strengthening these muscles can lead to better breathing control and endurance.

Reduced Risk of Respiratory Infections: Regular exercise can boost the immune system, making the body more resistant to respiratory infections.

Weight Management: Maintaining a healthy weight through exercise can reduce the strain on the respiratory system, particularly in seniors who may be prone to obesity-related respiratory issues.

Safe Exercise Tips for Seniors

Consult with a Healthcare Provider: Before starting any new exercise routine, seniors should consult with their healthcare provider to ensure that it's safe and appropriate for their individual health status.

Choose Low-Impact Activities: Low-impact exercises like walking, swimming, and stationary biking are gentle on the joints and are generally safe for seniors.

Warm-Up and Cool Down: Always begin and end exercise sessions with a warm-up and cool-down period to prevent muscle strains and injuries.

Listen to Your Body: Seniors should pay attention to how their bodies feel during exercise. If they experience pain, dizziness, or shortness of breath, they should stop immediately and seek medical advice if necessary.

Stay Hydrated: Proper hydration is essential during exercise to support lung function. Seniors should drink water before, during, and after physical activity.

Combining Breathing Exercises with Physical Activity

Integrating Breathing and Movement: Combining breathing exercises with physical activity can amplify the benefits of both practices. It enhances mindfulness, improves oxygenation, and promotes overall well-being. Here's how to synchronize breathing exercises with movement for enhanced benefits:

Conscious Breathing: Start by becoming aware of your breath. Pay attention to the natural rhythm of your breathing as you engage in physical activity. This awareness forms the foundation for combining the two practices.

Match Breath to Movement: Coordinate your breath with your physical movements. Inhale during the preparatory phase or when extending your body, and exhale during the exertion phase or when contracting your body. For example, during yoga, inhale as you raise your arms, and exhale as you fold forward.

Maintain a Smooth Flow: The goal is to create a seamless and smooth flow between your breath and movement. This synchronization promotes a sense of unity between body and mind.

Examples of Combined Practices

Walking and Breathing: While taking a brisk walk, synchronize your breath with your steps. Inhale for a certain number of steps, and exhale for the same number. This rhythmic breathing can enhance your walking experience and oxygenate your body effectively.

Yoga and Pranayama: Yoga is a prime example of combining movement and breath. Poses are often linked with specific breathing patterns. For instance, in the "Sun Salutation," each movement is accompanied by a breath, creating a harmonious flow.

Tai Chi and Deep Breathing: Tai Chi, known for its graceful and slow movements, is naturally paired with deep and mindful breathing. Inhale as you expand your posture, and exhale as you contract.

Stretching and Relaxation: Incorporate deep breathing during stretching exercises to release tension and increase flexibility. Inhale as you stretch, and exhale as you release the stretch.

By integrating breathing exercises with physical activity, seniors can elevate their exercise routine to a mindful and holistic practice. These combined practices not only enhance the benefits of both but also promote relaxation, reduce stress, and improve overall physical and mental well-being. This chapter will explore specific examples and guide seniors on how to seamlessly integrate these practices into their daily lives.

Dietary Adjustments for Specific Respiratory Conditions

Managing COPD and Asthma Through Diet: Diet plays a crucial role in managing respiratory conditions such as COPD and asthma. Here are some dietary considerations for seniors dealing with these conditions:

Anti-Inflammatory Foods: Both COPD and asthma involve inflammation of the airways. Consuming anti-inflammatory foods like fruits, vegetables, and whole grains can help reduce inflammation and ease symptoms. Berries, leafy greens, and nuts are rich in antioxidants that combat inflammation.

Omega-3 Fatty Acids: Foods high in omega-3 fatty acids, such as fatty fish (salmon, mackerel, trout), flaxseeds, and walnuts, have anti-inflammatory properties and can benefit lung health. Omega-3s may help reduce the frequency and severity of asthma attacks.

Vitamin D: Adequate vitamin D levels are essential for lung health. Seniors with respiratory conditions should ensure they get enough vitamin D from sources like fortified dairy products, fatty fish, and exposure to sunlight.

Magnesium: Magnesium-rich foods like spinach, almonds, and beans may help relax the airways and improve lung function, making them beneficial for managing asthma.

Fiber: High-fiber foods, including whole grains, legumes, and fruits, can support digestive health. Good digestion can reduce the pressure on the diaphragm and make breathing easier for individuals with respiratory conditions.

Avoiding Trigger Foods: Identifying and avoiding trigger foods is crucial for seniors with respiratory conditions. Common trigger foods can vary from person to person, but some general guidelines include:

Allergenic Foods: Seniors with asthma should be cautious of common food allergens like dairy, eggs, peanuts, tree nuts, soy, wheat, and fish. These allergens can sometimes exacerbate asthma symptoms.

Reflux-Inducing Foods: Gastroesophageal reflux disease (GERD) often coexists with respiratory conditions. Trigger foods for GERD, such as citrus fruits, tomatoes, spicy foods, and caffeine, can worsen acid reflux and respiratory symptoms.

Processed and High-Sodium Foods: Highly processed and high-sodium foods can contribute to inflammation and fluid retention, potentially making breathing more difficult.

Seniors should limit their intake of processed foods, canned soups, and excessive salt.

Gas-Producing Foods: Certain foods like beans, cabbage, and carbonated beverages can cause bloating and discomfort, which may affect breathing in individuals with respiratory conditions.

Individual Sensitivities: It's important for seniors to pay attention to their bodies and identify specific trigger foods that worsen their symptoms. Keeping a food diary can be helpful in this regard.

By making these dietary adjustments and avoiding trigger foods, seniors can take an active role in managing their respiratory conditions and improving their overall quality of life. This chapter will delve deeper into nutritional strategies tailored to specific needs, providing practical guidance for seniors to make informed dietary choices.

Overcoming Nutritional Challenges

Addressing Changes in Appetite: As seniors age, they often experience changes in appetite and metabolism. These changes can pose challenges to maintaining a healthy diet. Here are some tips for addressing these challenges:

Frequent, Smaller Meals: Seniors may find it more comfortable to eat smaller, more frequent meals throughout the day rather than three large meals. This approach can help maintain energy levels and support appetite.

Nutrient-Dense Snacking: opt for nutrient-dense snacks like Greek yogurt, mixed nuts, or whole-grain crackers with hummus. These snacks provide essential nutrients without excessive calories.

Hydration: Sometimes, thirst can be mistaken for hunger. Staying adequately hydrated can help regulate appetite. Drinking water or herbal teas throughout the day can be beneficial.

Flavorful Seasonings: Age-related changes in taste perception may lead to a reduced enjoyment of food. Using herbs, spices, and flavorful seasonings can make meals more appealing.

Consulting a Dietitian: If appetite changes are a significant concern, consulting a registered dietitian can provide personalized guidance to address specific nutritional needs.

Easy and Nutritious Meal Ideas

Preparing nutritious meals doesn't have to be complicated. Here are some simple meal ideas that are not only easy to prepare but also beneficial for lung health:

Vegetable Stir-Fry: Stir-frying a variety of colorful vegetables like bell peppers, broccoli, and carrots with lean protein (chicken, tofu, or shrimp) in a light, flavorful sauce is a quick and nutritious option.

Salmon Salad: Grilled or baked salmon served on a bed of mixed greens with a lemon vinaigrette is rich in omega-3 fatty acids and antioxidants.

Oatmeal with Berries: A bowl of oatmeal topped with fresh or frozen berries and a sprinkle of nuts or seeds is a fiber-rich breakfast that supports lung health.

Quinoa and Veggie Bowl: Cooked quinoa paired with sautéed spinach, cherry tomatoes, and chickpeas makes for a protein-packed, nutrient-dense meal.

Homemade Soup: Preparing a simple vegetable or chicken soup with plenty of vegetables and herbs provides both hydration and essential nutrients.

Smoothies: Blending fruits, leafy greens, yogurt, and a scoop of protein powder can create a satisfying and nutritious smoothie that's easy to consume.

Egg and Veggie Scramble: Scrambled eggs with sautéed spinach, tomatoes, and a sprinkle of cheese offer a protein boost and essential vitamins.

These meal ideas are not only easy to make but also provide the nutrients needed to support respiratory health. They can be adapted to individual preferences and dietary restrictions, making them suitable choices for seniors looking to enhance their lung function through nutrition.

The Impact of Weight on Respiratory Health

Understanding the Weight-Respiratory Connection: Maintaining a healthy weight is crucial for optimal respiratory health. Excess body weight, especially around the abdomen, can have a significant impact on the respiratory system. Here's how weight and respiratory health are interconnected:

Increased Workload: Excess weight puts additional pressure on the diaphragm and chest wall muscles. This increased workload can lead to shallow breathing and reduced lung capacity.

Obesity and Inflammation: Obesity is associated with chronic low-grade inflammation throughout the body, including the airways. This inflammation can exacerbate respiratory conditions like asthma and COPD.

Sleep Apnea: Obesity is a leading cause of obstructive sleep apnea, a condition where the airway becomes blocked during sleep, leading to interrupted breathing. Sleep apnea can significantly impact oxygen levels and overall respiratory health.

Reduced Lung Function: Studies have shown that obesity is linked to reduced lung function, making it harder to breathe efficiently.

Weight Management Strategies: Managing weight in a healthy, sustainable way is essential for seniors looking to improve their respiratory health. Here are some strategies to consider:

Balanced Diet: Focus on a balanced diet rich in whole foods, including fruits, vegetables, lean proteins, whole grains, and healthy fats. Portion control and mindful eating can help manage calorie intake.

Regular Physical Activity: Engage in regular physical activity suitable for your fitness level and health condition. Activities like walking, swimming, or gentle yoga can promote weight loss and improve lung function.

Consult a Healthcare Provider: If you have underlying health conditions or medications that may affect weight, consult your healthcare provider for personalized guidance.

Behavioral Changes: Address emotional eating or unhealthy eating patterns by seeking support from a therapist, counselor, or support group.

Stay Hydrated: Proper hydration is crucial for metabolism and overall health. Drinking water throughout the day can support weight management.

Sleep Quality: Prioritize good sleep hygiene to ensure restorative sleep, as poor sleep can contribute to weight gain.

Set Realistic Goals: Establish achievable weight loss goals to prevent frustration and promote long-term success.

Remember that weight management should be approached with patience and a focus on overall health rather than quick fixes. It's essential to consult with a healthcare provider or registered dietitian to develop a personalized plan that considers individual needs and any underlying medical conditions. Achieving and maintaining a healthy weight can significantly improve respiratory health and overall well-being for seniors.

The Role of Supplements in Respiratory Health

When Supplements Are Beneficial: Supplements can play a role in supporting respiratory health, especially for seniors who may have specific dietary or health needs. Here are some situations when supplements may be beneficial:

Vitamin D: Seniors often have lower exposure to sunlight, which is essential for the body's synthesis of vitamin D. Vitamin D is crucial for immune function and can support respiratory health. Supplements may be recommended for those with vitamin D deficiency.

Omega-3 Fatty Acids: Omega-3 fatty acids, found in fish oil supplements, have anti-inflammatory properties, and can help reduce inflammation in the airways. They may be beneficial for individuals with respiratory conditions like asthma.

Antioxidants: Antioxidants like vitamin C and vitamin E can help protect lung tissue from oxidative stress and inflammation. These supplements may be considered for individuals at risk of respiratory conditions or those with increased exposure to environmental pollutants.

Herbal Supplements: Some herbal supplements, such as turmeric or ginger, have anti-inflammatory properties and can support overall lung function. However, it's essential to consult with a healthcare provider before using herbal supplements, as they can interact with medications.

Consulting Healthcare Professionals: Before starting any supplements, it's crucial to consult with healthcare professionals, including your primary care physician or a registered dietitian. Here's why professional guidance is essential:

Personalized Assessment: Healthcare providers can assess your individual health status, dietary intake, and potential deficiencies. They can determine whether supplements are necessary and recommend specific ones based on your needs.

Medication Interactions: Some supplements can interact with medications, affecting their effectiveness or causing adverse effects. Healthcare professionals can review your medications and ensure there are no contraindications.

Proper Dosage: Healthcare providers can recommend the appropriate dosage of supplements to avoid overconsumption, which can lead to adverse effects.

Monitoring and Adjustments: Regular monitoring of supplement use is essential to assess their effectiveness and make any necessary adjustments to the regimen.

Safety: Healthcare professionals can ensure that the chosen supplements are safe for your age, health status, and any underlying medical conditions.

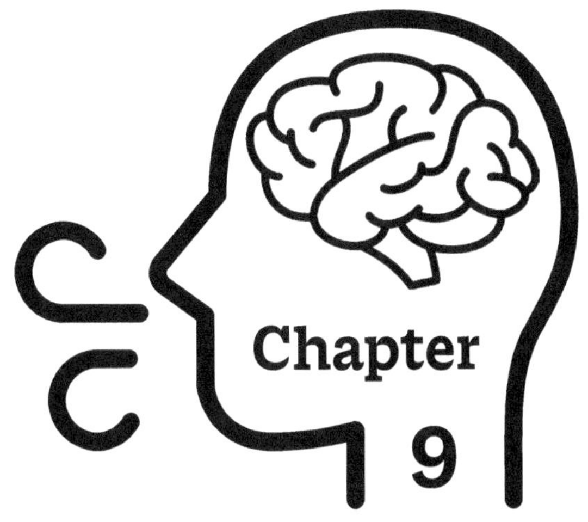

CULTIVATING MENTAL CLARITY THROUGH MINDFUL BREATHING

With a relaxed breath, let your mind wander to a peaceful bamboo sanctuary, where the gentle ripple of water and the soothing chorus of birds instill a sense of serenity, guiding you into a mindful space, prepared to absorb the life-affirming lessons of breath and awareness in this chapter.

Uniting the Mind and Breath

In Chapter 9, we delve into the profound synergy between mindfulness and breathing exercises, illuminating the path to improved mental clarity and emotional equilibrium for seniors.

This chapter is dedicated to harnessing the power of mindful breathing as a transformative tool for mental well-being.

Connecting Mind and Breath: The art of mindful breathing entails a profound connection between the mind and breath. It's about becoming acutely aware of each breath, each moment, and each sensation. This chapter introduces seniors to this transformative practice, highlighting how the simple act of paying attention to their breath can be a gateway to enhanced mental clarity and emotional harmony.

The primary goal of this chapter is to empower seniors with the knowledge and techniques necessary to incorporate mindfulness into their daily lives. By doing so, they can reap the benefits of mental clarity, reduced stress, and emotional balance. The chapter will equip seniors with practical mindfulness exercises that can be seamlessly integrated with breathing techniques.

As we explore the depths of mindfulness and breathing in the pages that follow, seniors will discover that they possess the tools to navigate the complexities of the mind. By bringing mindfulness to their breath, they can anchor themselves in the present moment, cultivate mental clarity, and nurture emotional resilience. This chapter invites seniors on a journey inward, where the simple act of mindful breathing can illuminate the path to a more balanced and centered existence.

Understanding Mindfulness: A Path to Present-Moment Awareness

In this section, we delve into the essence of mindfulness, shedding light on its fundamental principles and elucidating the profound benefits it offers to seniors.

Basics of Mindfulness: Mindfulness is a practice rooted in the art of being fully present in the moment, without judgment or distraction. It involves cultivating a heightened awareness of one's thoughts, emotions, bodily sensations, and surroundings. The core principles of mindfulness revolve around:

Present-Moment Awareness: Mindfulness encourages individuals to embrace the here and now, anchoring their attention to the current moment rather than dwelling on the past or worrying about the future. This practice helps seniors appreciate the richness of each moment, fostering a sense of fulfillment and contentment.

Non-Judgmental Observation: Mindfulness invites individuals to observe their thoughts and feelings without criticism or attachment. It's about acknowledging the thoughts and emotions that arise without labeling them as "good" or "bad." This non-judgmental stance empowers seniors to navigate their inner landscapes with compassion and self-acceptance.

Benefits of Mindfulness for Seniors: For seniors, mindfulness holds immense promise as a tool for enhancing overall well-being.

Here are some of the key benefits:

Stress Reduction: Mindfulness practices, such as mindful breathing, enable seniors to manage stress more effectively. By remaining present and non-reactive in the face of stressors, seniors can reduce their perceived stress levels and develop healthier coping mechanisms.

Improved Mood: Mindfulness fosters emotional regulation and resilience. Seniors who engage in mindfulness often report improved mood, reduced symptoms of anxiety and depression, and a greater sense of emotional stability.

Enhanced Cognitive Function: Mindfulness exercises can sharpen cognitive function, including memory, attention, and problem-solving skills. This is particularly valuable for seniors seeking to maintain mental sharpness as they age.

Incorporating mindfulness into daily life can be a transformative journey for seniors. It empowers them to savor the present, navigate life's challenges with grace, and cultivate a deeper understanding of themselves. The union of mindfulness and breathing exercises in the chapters to come offers seniors a comprehensive toolkit for holistic well-being.

The Link Between Breathing and Mindfulness: A Path to Inner Calm

In this section, we explore the profound connection between conscious breathing and mindfulness, shedding light on how the simple act of focusing on one's breath can serve as a gateway to a mindful state of being. Additionally, we delve into scientific insights that substantiate the benefits of mindful breathing, particularly for seniors.

Breath as a Tool for Mindfulness: Conscious and deliberate breathing is at the heart of mindfulness practices. The breath serves as a powerful anchor to the present moment. Here's how it works:

Focusing Attention: When individuals turn their attention to the rhythm of their breath, they shift their focus from the whirlwind of thoughts and worries to the immediate physical experience of breathing. This redirection of attention acts as a reset button for the mind, allowing it to disengage from distractions and settle into the here and now.

Cultivating Awareness: Mindful breathing entails observing the breath without judgment. Seniors are encouraged to notice the gentle rise and fall of their chest or the sensation of the breath passing through their nostrils. This heightened awareness of bodily sensations promotes a profound sense of presence.

Reducing Stress: As seniors engage in mindful breathing, they learn to regulate their breath, slowing it down and making it deeper. This deliberate breath control triggers the body's relaxation response, reducing stress hormones and promoting a state of calm.

Scientific Insights:

Stress Reduction: Numerous studies have shown that mindful breathing techniques can significantly reduce stress levels in seniors. This is particularly pertinent as chronic stress can exacerbate various health issues, including respiratory conditions.

Improved Cognitive Function: Research suggests that regular mindfulness practices, including mindful breathing, can enhance cognitive function and memory, which is valuable for seniors looking to maintain mental acuity.

Emotional Well-being: Seniors who engage in mindful breathing often report improved emotional well-being, including reduced symptoms of anxiety and depression. This highlights the positive impact of mindfulness on mental health in the senior population.

Incorporating mindful breathing into daily life equips seniors with a potent tool for managing stress, enhancing cognitive function, and fostering emotional balance. It aligns perfectly with the holistic approach to well-being advocated in this guide, providing seniors with the means to nurture both their respiratory and mental health.

Mindful Breathing Techniques: Cultivating Presence and Focus

Mindful Observation of Breath: This foundational technique invites seniors to simply observe their natural breath without any intention to change it. Here's how to guide readers through this practice:

Find a Quiet Space: Begin by finding a quiet and comfortable space where you won't be disturbed. Sit in a chair or on the floor with your back straight but not rigid.

Close Your Eyes: Gently close your eyes or soften your gaze if closing your eyes isn't comfortable for you.

Focus on Your Breath: Bring your attention to your breath. Feel the sensation of the breath as it enters and leaves your nostrils or the rise and fall of your chest or abdomen.

Observe Without Judgment: As you breathe, observe your breath without judgment. Notice the rhythm, depth, and texture of your breath. Be fully present with each inhale and exhale.

Gentle Redirect: If your mind starts to wander (as it naturally does), gently redirect your focus back to your breath. There's no need to criticize yourself for drifting; it's a normal part of the practice.

This technique is a profound way to ground oneself in the present moment, fostering a sense of inner calm and reducing mental chatter.

Counting Breaths for Focus: Counting breaths is an effective method to maintain focus during mindful breathing. Here's how to introduce this technique:

Choose a Count: Decide on a count that works for you, such as counting to four or five with each inhale and exhale.

Begin the Practice: Start by inhaling slowly while silently counting "one." Then exhale slowly while counting "two." Continue this pattern, counting to your chosen number.

Start Over: Once you reach your chosen count, start over from "one." If you lose count or become distracted, gently return to "one" and begin again.

Counting breaths provides a structured way to anchor your attention to the breath, enhancing your ability to stay present and focused.

These mindful breathing techniques are valuable tools for seniors to cultivate mindfulness, improve mental clarity, and reduce stress. They can be practiced anytime and anywhere, making them accessible for daily use in various situations.

Integrating Mindfulness into Breathing Exercises: A Path to Enhanced Mental Clarity

Integrating mindfulness into the breathing exercises introduced in previous chapters can elevate their effectiveness and contribute to enhanced mental clarity and emotional well-being. Here's how seniors can combine these practices:

Mindfulness in Diaphragmatic Breathing: When practicing diaphragmatic breathing, seniors can infuse mindfulness by paying close attention to the sensations associated with each breath. As they inhale deeply, they can focus on the expansion of the abdomen, feeling the rise and fall with each breath. This heightened awareness of the physical sensations connects the breath to the present moment, fostering mindfulness.

Mindful Pursed-Lip Breathing: Pursed-lip breathing, known for its calming effect, can be further enhanced with mindfulness. Seniors can focus on the slow and deliberate exhale, observing the gentle release of tension. This mindful approach aids in stress reduction and encourages relaxation.

Coordinated Breathing with Mindfulness: During coordinated breathing exercises, seniors can combine the rhythm of their breath with mindful counting. For instance, they can count to four during the inhale and count to six during the exhale. This not only enhances focus but also encourages a sense of control over the breath, promoting emotional balance.

Establishing a Routine Practice: To maximize the benefits of mindful breathing, seniors are encouraged to establish a routine practice. Consistency is key to experiencing the profound effects of mindfulness on mental clarity. Setting aside dedicated time each day, whether in the morning, during a break, or before bedtime, allows seniors to cultivate mindfulness as a habit.

By integrating mindfulness into their breathing exercises and maintaining a regular practice, seniors can enjoy a deeper sense of mental clarity, improved emotional balance, and a heightened connection to the present moment. This combination of breath and mindfulness becomes a powerful tool for enhancing overall well-being and achieving a sense of inner peace.

Mindfulness for Emotional Regulation: A Path to Inner Peace

Mindfulness, when integrated into breathing exercises, serves as a valuable tool for emotional regulation, helping seniors manage stress, anxiety, depression, and loneliness. Here are specific practices for each:

Managing Stress and Anxiety: Mindful breathing techniques like "Mindful Observation of Breath" and "Counting Breaths for Focus" can be highly effective for managing stress and anxiety.

Seniors can start by finding a quiet space, sitting comfortably, and bringing their attention to the sensation of each breath. As they inhale and exhale, they can observe the natural flow of breath without judgment. By counting breaths or focusing on the rise and fall of the abdomen, they anchor their awareness to the present moment, reducing the grip of anxious or stressful thoughts.

Coping with Depression and Loneliness: For seniors dealing with depression or feelings of loneliness, mindful walking meditation can be immensely beneficial. This practice involves walking slowly and mindfully, paying attention to each step and the sensations in the body. Seniors can take this practice outdoors and connect with nature, further enhancing their emotional well-being. Additionally, practicing loving-kindness meditation, where they send wishes of happiness and well-being to themselves and others, can counter feelings of loneliness and foster a sense of connection.

Mindful breathing practices provide seniors with a way to cultivate emotional resilience and inner peace. By incorporating these techniques into their daily routine, they can gradually experience a shift in their emotional well-being. As they develop a deeper connection to the present moment and their inner selves, they are better equipped to navigate life's challenges with clarity and a greater sense of emotional balance.

Overcoming Common Challenges in Mindful Breathing

Dealing with a Wandering Mind: It's common for the mind to wander during mindfulness and breathing exercises, especially for seniors who may have busy thoughts. To address this challenge, seniors can employ several strategies:

Gentle Redirecting: Instead of chastising themselves for a wandering mind, seniors should practice gentle redirection. When they notice their thoughts have strayed, they can kindly bring their attention back to the breath without judgment. This approach fosters self-compassion and patience.

Use of Anchors: Seniors can utilize anchors to tether their focus to the present moment. These anchors can be physical sensations, such as the feeling of the breath entering and leaving the nostrils, the rise and fall of the abdomen, or the sensation of their feet touching the ground during walking meditation. Anchors provide a point of concentration and reduce distractions.

Counting Breaths: Counting breaths can serve as a useful technique to maintain focus. For instance, they can count each inhale and exhale up to a specific number (e.g., five) and then start again. This rhythmic counting helps center their attention on the breath.

Adapting Practices for Physical Limitations: Physical limitations or health issues can pose challenges to traditional mindfulness practices. To make these practices more accessible, seniors can consider the following adaptations:

Seated or Supported Postures: Seniors with mobility issues can practice mindfulness and breathing exercises while seated in a comfortable chair or on a cushion. Using a chair with good back support or sitting against a wall can provide added stability.

Gentle Movements: For those with limited mobility, incorporating gentle movements, such as hand or arm stretches, into their mindful breathing practice can enhance the experience. These movements promote circulation and reduce stiffness.

Mindful Listening: Seniors who find it challenging to focus on the breath due to physical discomfort can explore mindful listening. This involves paying close attention to sounds in the environment, which can serve as an alternative anchor for mindfulness.

Embracing Mindfulness in Daily Life

Mindful Eating: Encourage seniors to savor their meals by eating slowly and paying full attention to the flavors, textures, and smells of their food. This practice not only enhances the dining experience but also promotes better digestion.

Mindful Walking: Whether indoors or outdoors, suggest that seniors take mindful walks. They can focus on the sensation of each step, the movement of their body, and the sounds of nature or the environment. This practice helps clear the mind and reduce stress.

Mindful Chores: Turning routine chores into mindful activities can be transformative. For example, while washing dishes, they can immerse themselves fully in the process, feeling the warm water, noticing the soap bubbles, and appreciating the cleanliness of each dish.

Creating Mindful Moments: In addition to incorporating mindfulness into specific activities, seniors can create mindful moments throughout the day:

Breathing Breaks: Recommend taking short breaks during the day to practice mindful breathing. These breaks can be as brief as a few deep breaths. Seniors can pause before or after tasks to center themselves and regain mental clarity.

Transition Mindfulness: Encourage mindfulness during transitions between activities. When switching from one task to another, seniors can take a moment to focus on their breath, calming their mind before moving on.

Nature Connection: If possible, spending time in nature can be inherently mindful. Seniors can take leisurely strolls in a park, garden, or natural setting, immersing themselves in the sights, sounds, and sensations of the environment.

By weaving mindfulness into their daily lives, seniors can experience improved mental clarity, reduced stress, and a deeper connection to the present moment. These practices not only enhance their overall well-being but also make mindfulness an integral part of their daily routines.

Exploring Advanced Mindful Breathing Practices

The long history of yoga breathing exercises, developed in the ancient tradition of India, stands in stark contrast to the relatively recent adoption of mindfulness practices in Western cultures. Yoga has incorporated these breathing exercises for thousands of years as a fundamental component of physical and mental well-being. These practices, often referred to as pranayama, are deeply ingrained in yogic philosophy and have been refined over centuries within the Eastern tradition. In contrast, mindfulness practices, including various forms of meditation and mindful breathing, have gained popularity in Western cultures primarily in the last few decades. While yoga and mindfulness share commonalities in their emphasis on breath awareness, the advanced mindful breathing practices offered to seniors build upon this rich history, drawing from both Eastern and Western traditions to deepen their mindfulness journey.

For seniors who have embraced mindfulness and wish to deepen their practice, there are advanced techniques and resources available:

Deepening the Practice

Body Scan Meditation: This advanced practice involves systematically scanning the body from head to toe, focusing on each body part and observing sensations without judgment. It enhances awareness of bodily sensations and can be deeply relaxing.

Insight Meditation: Insight Meditation, also known as Vipassana in the Buddhist tradition, is a meditation technique that involves observing the breath and bodily sensations with a heightened level of awareness. It aims to develop insight into the impermanent nature of sensations and the nature of the mind.

Loving-Kindness Meditation: Also known as Metta meditation in the Buddhist tradition, involves sending wishes of love, compassion, and well-being to oneself and others. It fosters feelings of kindness and connection, making it an advanced form of mindfulness.

Guided Meditations:

Online Resources: There are numerous websites and apps that offer guided mindfulness and mindful breathing meditations. Some popular platforms include Insight Timer, Headspace, and Calm. These guided sessions can provide structure and support for advanced practice.

Yoga and Meditation Classes: Seniors can consider joining local yoga or meditation classes that offer guidance on advanced mindful breathing techniques. Instructors can provide personalized instruction and feedback.

Books and Audio Programs: Many authors and mindfulness experts have published books and audio programs that delve into advanced mindfulness practices. These resources can be valuable companions on the journey to deepening mindfulness.

It's important to emphasize that advanced mindfulness practices require patience and consistency. Seniors should progress at their own pace, and it's perfectly acceptable to continue with simpler practices if they find them more suitable. The goal is not perfection but a gradual deepening of awareness and presence in each moment. Advanced practices can provide a profound sense of inner peace, emotional resilience, and clarity of mind for those who explore them.

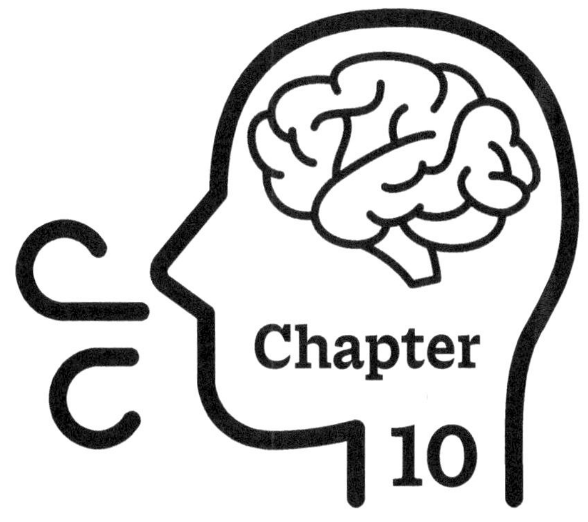

SUCCESS STORIES AND FURTHER EXPLORATION

With a relaxed breath, let your mind wander to a peaceful bamboo sanctuary, where the gentle ripple of water and the soothing chorus of birds instill a sense of serenity, guiding you into a mindful space, prepared to absorb the life-affirming lessons of breath and awareness in this chapter.

Drawing Inspiration from Real-Life Stories

Welcome to the final chapter of our journey – a chapter filled with inspiration, hope, and the real-life stories of seniors who have experienced the transformative power of breathing exercises. As we delve into these narratives, you'll witness firsthand the incredible impact that intentional and mindful breathing can have on the lives of older adults.

The Heartwarming Stories of Seniors

Each story in this chapter is a testament to resilience, determination, and the potential for growth, no matter one's age. You'll read about individuals who, despite facing various challenges, embraced the practice of breathing exercises and reaped the rewards.

From Joe, a retired teacher who overcame chronic stress and anxiety to find inner peace through daily mindful breathing, to Mary, a grandmother who discovered newfound energy and zest for life by combining breathing exercises with gentle yoga – these stories serve as beacons of hope and motivation.

Joe's Journey to Tranquility

Joe, a retired teacher, had spent years battling chronic stress and anxiety. Sleepless nights and a racing mind had become his norm. However, Joe decided to take control of his mental health through breathing exercises. With consistent daily practice, he noticed a significant reduction in stress levels. His anxiety began to dissipate, replaced by a profound sense of inner peace. Joe's story reminds us that, no matter our age, we have the capacity to find serenity through the breath.

Mary's Reinvigoration Through Breath and Yoga

Mary, a loving grandmother, was struggling with age-related fatigue and a sense of physical stagnation. She embarked on a journey that combined breathing exercises with gentle yoga. Over time, she felt a surge of energy and vitality coursing through her body. Mary's story exemplifies the incredible synergy between breath and movement, proving that seniors can experience a rejuvenation of body and spirit through these practices.

Tom's Triumph Over Respiratory Challenges

Tom, a retired engineer, had been living with chronic obstructive pulmonary disease (COPD). Breathing had become a daily struggle, limiting his ability to enjoy life fully. Through targeted breathing exercises for COPD, Tom experienced improved lung function and a newfound sense of control over his breath. His story showcases the potential for seniors with respiratory conditions to regain hope and vitality.

Sarah's Serenity in Mindful Moments

Sarah, a senior who had faced her share of life's challenges, discovered the power of mindfulness and breath. By weaving mindful breathing into her daily life, she found a sense of emotional balance she hadn't felt in years. Sarah's story highlights the profound impact that mindfulness can have on emotional well-being, demonstrating that seniors can experience increased inner calm and resilience.

These diverse and heartwarming stories serve as beacons of hope and motivation for seniors and caregivers alike. They remind us that the journey of well-being and self-discovery continues throughout our lives, and the breath is a powerful ally on that path. May these testimonials inspire you to embark on your own transformative journey with breathing exercises.

Analyzing the Impact of Breathing Exercises

The impact of breathing exercises on seniors' lives is profound and multifaceted. Through a collection of stories, we delve into the tangible physical improvements and the mental and emotional benefits that have resulted from the consistent practice of breathing exercises.

Physical Improvements

Enhanced Respiratory Function

One common theme among our success stories is the remarkable improvement in respiratory function. Many seniors, like Tom, who battled conditions such as COPD, have experienced a significant increase in lung capacity and ease of breathing. These stories highlight the potential for breathing exercises to empower seniors with respiratory conditions to regain control over their breath and enjoy a higher quality of life.

Vitality and Energy

Stories like Mary's illustrate how breathing exercises, when combined with movement, can infuse seniors with a renewed sense of vitality and energy. Seniors who were once plagued by fatigue found themselves embracing life with newfound enthusiasm. This physical reinvigoration has allowed them to engage in activities they had previously thought were beyond their reach.

Mental and Emotional Benefits
Stress Reduction

The mental and emotional benefits of breathing exercises cannot be overstated. Testimonials from individuals like Joe demonstrate how daily practice can lead to a substantial reduction in stress and anxiety levels. The breath becomes a reliable anchor in times of turbulence, fostering a sense of calm and serenity.

Emotional Resilience

Stories like Sarah's emphasize how mindfulness and breath work hand in hand to bolster emotional resilience. Seniors have reported feeling better equipped to cope with life's challenges, including feelings of loneliness and depression. Through mindful breathing, they have found a sanctuary of emotional stability and inner strength.

These success stories collectively reveal the transformative potential of breathing exercises. They underscore the fact that age should never be a barrier to improving physical health and enhancing mental and emotional well-being. Seniors who have embraced breathing practices have not only extended their vitality but have also discovered the profound capacity of the breath to enrich and uplift their lives.

Lessons Learned from Real-Life Experiences

The success stories of seniors who have embraced breathing exercises reveal valuable insights and common themes that can inspire and guide others on their journey to better respiratory health and well-being.

Common Themes and Takeaways

Consistency is Key

One consistent theme across these stories is the importance of regular, consistent practice. Seniors who experienced the most significant improvements in their physical, mental, and emotional well-being were those who committed to daily or near-daily breathing exercises. This highlights the notion that real progress is built upon a foundation of dedication and routine.

Mindful Awareness

Another crucial takeaway is the power of mindful awareness. Many seniors stressed the significance of being present in the moment while practicing breathing exercises. Mindful breathing not only enhances the effectiveness of the exercises but also fosters a sense of inner calm and mental clarity.

Adaptability and Patience

These stories also teach us about adaptability and patience. Seniors who faced physical limitations or health challenges found ways to modify exercises to suit their needs. This adaptability, coupled with patience, allowed them to gradually progress and experience positive changes over time.

Tips and Strategies

Start Small and Build

For those just beginning their journey with breathing exercises, the stories advise starting small and gradually building up. Begin with simple techniques like diaphragmatic breathing and gradually explore more advanced practices as confidence and comfort levels grow.

Seek Support and Guidance

Several seniors emphasized the importance of seeking support and guidance. Whether through joining a local group or working with a qualified instructor, having a support system in place can provide motivation, encouragement, and the opportunity to learn from others.

Track Progress

Many success stories noted the benefits of keeping a journal to track progress. Documenting one's experiences, physical improvements, and emotional changes can be motivating and help individuals stay committed to their practice.

In conclusion, these real-life experiences of seniors who have embraced breathing exercises teach us that consistency, mindfulness, adaptability, and patience are key to success. By starting small, seeking support, and tracking progress, anyone can embark on a journey to better respiratory health and overall well-being, no matter their age or previous experience with breathing exercises.

The Role of Community and Support

In the journey of incorporating breathing exercises into one's daily life, the role of community and support cannot be underestimated. For seniors, finding support in groups, whether in-person or online, can be a game-changer in terms of motivation, accountability, and shared learning.

Finding Support in Groups

Many seniors have found solace and encouragement by joining breathing exercise groups or participating in online forums dedicated to respiratory health and well-being. These communities provide a safe space for individuals to share their experiences, challenges, and successes. It's in these groups that seniors often discover that they are not alone in their pursuit of better respiratory health.

Encouraging Group Practice

Practicing breathing exercises in a group setting offers unique benefits, especially for seniors.

Here are some reasons why group practice is so valuable:

Motivation and Accountability

In a group, there's a natural sense of accountability. Seniors are more likely to stay committed to their breathing exercise routines when they know that others are relying on them. The collective energy of the group can boost motivation and make it easier to establish and maintain a regular practice.

Shared Learning

Within a group, individuals can learn from each other's experiences and insights. Seniors may discover new techniques or approaches to breathing exercises that they hadn't considered on their own. This shared knowledge can enrich their practice and lead to more profound benefits.

Emotional Support

Breathing exercise groups also provide emotional support. Seniors can openly discuss any challenges they face, whether related to their health or their practice, and receive empathy and encouragement from their peers.

Social Connection

Participating in group practice fosters social connections, which are essential for overall well-being, especially in later life. Seniors can build friendships and enjoy the camaraderie of like-minded individuals.

In summary, the role of community and support in the journey of integrating breathing exercises into daily life cannot be overstated. Whether through joining local groups or connecting with others online, seniors can find motivation, shared learning, emotional support, and valuable social connections that enhance their respiratory health and overall quality of life.

Resources for Further Learning

As seniors embark on their journey to explore breathing exercises and enhance their respiratory health, there are numerous resources available to support their quest for knowledge and well-being. Here are some valuable resources to consider:

Books and Online Resources

"Breath: The New Science of a Lost Art" by James Nestor: This bestselling book delves into the science and history of breathing, offering insights into how proper breathing can transform health.

"The Healing Power of the Breath" by Richard P. Brown and Patricia L. Gerbarg: This book explores the connection between breath and health, providing practical exercises for relaxation and stress reduction.

Local and Online Resources

Online Articles and Blogs: There are several reputable websites and blogs dedicated to respiratory health and breathing exercises. Look for articles that provide guidance on different techniques and their benefits.

YouTube: YouTube is a treasure trove of instructional videos on breathing exercises. Many yoga and wellness instructors offer free tutorials on various techniques.

Local Community Centers: Check with local community centers, senior centers, or fitness studios for classes specifically designed for seniors. These may include yoga, tai chi, or meditation classes that incorporate breathing exercises.

Online Learning Platforms: Websites like Udemy, Coursera, and Skillshare offer a wide range of online courses, including those focused on breathing techniques and mindfulness. Look for courses that cater to seniors.

Yoga and Meditation Apps: There are numerous apps available for smartphones and tablets that provide guided sessions for breathing exercises, meditation, and yoga. Some popular options include Headspace, Calm, and Yoga for Seniors.

Virtual Workshops: Keep an eye out for virtual workshops and webinars conducted by experts in the field of respiratory health and mindfulness. These events often provide in-depth knowledge and interactive sessions.

Local Yoga Studios: Many yoga studios offer classes tailored to seniors. These classes typically incorporate breathing exercises, gentle movements, and relaxation techniques.

When seeking out resources, it's essential to choose those that align with personal preferences and goals. Whether through books, online platforms, local classes, or virtual workshops, seniors have a wealth of options to continue their exploration of breathing exercises and respiratory health. These resources can be valuable companions on the journey toward improved well-being and a deeper understanding of the mind-breath connection.

Encouraging Lifelong Learning and Practice

As we conclude this comprehensive guide on breathing exercises for seniors, it's essential to emphasize that the journey of exploring and benefiting from these practices is not finite; it's a lifelong voyage filled with continuous learning and self-discovery. Here are some key points to inspire readers to embrace breathing exercises as an enduring part of their lives:

The Journey Ahead

Breathing exercises are not merely a set of techniques but a path towards enhanced well-being and self-awareness. As you've discovered in this guide, conscious breathing can positively impact physical health, mental clarity, emotional balance, and overall quality of life. However, it's important to recognize that the benefits of these practices accrue over time.

Consider this journey as an ongoing process, much like tending to a garden. Just as a garden will flourish with consistent care, your practice of breathing exercises will thrive with regular attention. The positive changes you've experienced are just the beginning; there's so much more to explore and gain as you continue down this path.

Staying Curious and Open-Minded

One of the most beautiful aspects of the world of breathing exercises is its vastness and diversity. There are countless techniques, traditions, and philosophies to explore. As you progress on your journey, remain curious and open-minded. Don't hesitate to try new practices, attend workshops, or seek guidance from experienced instructors.

Embrace the idea that there is always more to discover about yourself and your breath. Each practice, whether it's a simple mindfulness exercise or an advanced Pranayama technique, offers a unique perspective and potential for growth. Be willing to adapt and evolve your practice as you gain insights and as your needs change over time.

Remember that your breathing journey is a personal one, and there is no one-size-fits-all approach. Your practice can reflect your individuality and a means of self-expression.

We've learned that breathing exercises are a versatile tool with the power to:

Enhance Respiratory Health: Breathing exercises can strengthen the respiratory system, improve lung function, and provide relief from conditions such as COPD and asthma.

Cultivate Mindfulness: Mindful breathing fosters present-moment awareness, reduces stress, and enhances cognitive function, offering mental and emotional clarity.

Energize and Relax: By combining rhythmic and energizing techniques, seniors can strike a balance between relaxation and vitality, ensuring a holistic approach to well-being.

Be Adapted for Individual Needs: Breathing exercises can be tailored to accommodate physical limitations and health concerns, ensuring accessibility for all.

Tips for Safe Practice

Safety is paramount when practicing breathing exercises, especially for seniors. Here are some essential tips to ensure a safe and beneficial experience:

Safety Guidelines:

Start Slowly: Begin with simple and gentle breathing exercises, especially if you are new to this practice. Gradually increase the complexity and duration as you become more comfortable.

Pay Attention to Body Signals: Listen to your body. If you experience pain, discomfort, dizziness, or shortness of breath during any exercise, stop immediately and seek medical advice if needed.

Choose a Comfortable Environment: Practice in a quiet, well-ventilated space free from distractions. Use a comfortable chair or cushion to sit on or lie down if preferred.

Maintain Proper Posture: Sit or stand with good posture. If sitting, ensure your feet are flat on the floor, and your back is supported. Good posture enhances the effectiveness of breathing exercises.

Stay Hydrated: Proper hydration supports lung function. Drink water throughout the day to keep your respiratory system functioning optimally.

Avoid Overexertion: Don't push yourself too hard. Breathing exercises should be relaxing, not strenuous. Overexertion can lead to fatigue and discomfort.

When to Consult a Professional:

Existing Health Conditions: If you have pre-existing respiratory conditions like chronic obstructive pulmonary disease (COPD), asthma, or heart disease, consult your healthcare provider before starting any new breathing exercise routine.

Recent Surgery: If you've had recent surgery, especially on your chest or abdomen, consult your surgeon or physician before engaging in breathing exercises that involve deep or forceful inhalation or exhalation.

Medication Changes: If you've recently started or changed medications, inform your healthcare provider. Some medications may affect your respiratory response to exercise.

Dizziness or Fainting Episodes: If you've experienced unexplained dizziness, fainting, or loss of consciousness, consult a healthcare professional to rule out any underlying medical issues.

Severe Shortness of Breath: If you experience severe shortness of breath, especially at rest, seek immediate medical attention. It could be a sign of a medical emergency.

Remember that safety should always come first when practicing breathing exercises. If in doubt, consult a qualified healthcare professional who can provide personalized guidance and ensure that your practice aligns with your specific health needs and conditions.

Enhancing the Effectiveness of Breathing Exercises

To maximize the benefits of breathing exercises, it's essential to optimize your practice. Here are some tips to help you make the most of your breathing exercises:

Optimizing Practice:

Choose the Right Time: Find a time that works best for you. Some people prefer to practice breathing exercises in the morning to start the day refreshed, while others find it helpful to unwind with these exercises in the evening. Experiment to determine when you feel most relaxed and focused.

Create an Ideal Environment: Select a peaceful and comfortable space for your practice. It should be free from distractions and have good ventilation. Dim lighting and soothing background music or nature sounds can enhance the ambiance.

Combine with Meditation: Consider incorporating meditation into your routine. Combining mindful breathing with meditation can deepen your practice and promote mental clarity and emotional balance.

Explore Guided Practices: Utilize guided breathing exercises and meditation apps or recordings. These resources can provide structured and immersive experiences, especially beneficial for beginners.

Progress and Adaptation:

Monitor Your Progress: Keep a journal to record your experiences and track your progress. Note any changes in your breathing, energy levels, and overall well-being. This helps you gauge the effectiveness of your practice.

Adapt to Your Needs: As you become more proficient, don't hesitate to adapt your exercises. You can increase the duration or complexity of your breathing techniques to continue challenging yourself. However, always do so gradually and comfortably.

Consider Health Changes: If your health condition changes or if you experience new symptoms, consult a healthcare professional to adjust your breathing exercises accordingly. Adapt the exercises to accommodate your current health status.

Set Realistic Goals: Define clear and achievable goals for your practice. Whether it's reducing stress, improving lung function, or enhancing mindfulness, having specific objectives can help you stay motivated and track your progress.

Stay Consistent: Consistency is key to reaping the long-term benefits of breathing exercises. Aim to practice regularly, even if it's just for a few minutes each day. Over time, your efforts will accumulate, leading to lasting improvements in your respiratory health and overall well-being.

Overcoming Common Challenges:

Distractions: It's natural for your mind to wander during practice. When distractions arise, acknowledge them without judgment and gently guide your focus back to your breath. Over time, this skill will improve, enhancing your ability to concentrate.

Restlessness or Impatience: If you find it challenging to sit still or feel impatient with the pace of your progress, remind yourself that patience is an essential part of the practice. Experiment with shorter sessions initially and gradually extend them as you become more comfortable.

Physical Discomfort: Seniors may experience discomfort due to age-related conditions. Modify your practice to accommodate any physical limitations. You can practice breathing exercises while sitting in a comfortable chair or even lying down. Ensure your body is well-supported to reduce strain.

Inconsistency: Maintaining a consistent practice can be challenging. Establish a daily routine and integrate breathing exercises into your daily activities. Set reminders or practice at the same time each day to build a habit.

Lack of Motivation: Motivation can wane, especially during plateaus. Remind yourself of the benefits you've experienced so far and set new goals. Joining a community group or class can provide external motivation and support.

Dealing with Plateaus:

Stay Patient: Plateaus are a natural part of any practice. Understand that progress is not always linear. Instead of getting discouraged, focus on maintaining your practice consistently.

Explore Advanced Techniques: Plateaus can be an opportunity to explore more advanced breathing techniques. These can challenge you in new ways and reignite your interest in the practice.

Mindful Reflection: Use plateaus as an opportunity for introspection and self-discovery. Reflect on your practice, its impact on your life, and any changes you'd like to make.

Seek Guidance: Consult with a qualified instructor or health-care professional if you're stuck at a plateau. They can provide personalized guidance and suggest modifications to your practice.

Celebrate Small Wins: Even if you're not making rapid progress, celebrate small victories along the way. Notice any subtle improvements in your breathing, stress levels, or overall well-being.

Recommended Reading and Websites:

Books: There are several comprehensive books about breathing exercises and respiratory health. Some notable titles include "The Healing Power of the Breath" by Richard P. Brown and Patricia L. Gerbarg, "Breath: The New Science of a Lost Art" by James Nestor, and "Yoga Anatomy" by Leslie Kaminoff and Amy Matthews.

Websites: Explore reputable websites dedicated to respiratory health and wellness. Websites like the American Lung Association (lung.org), Mayo Clinic (mayoclinic.org), and Harvard Health Publishing (health.harvard.edu) offer informative articles, research updates, and practical advice.

Online Courses: Consider enrolling in online courses or workshops related to breathing exercises and mindfulness. Platforms like Coursera, Udemy, and Mindful.org offer courses led by experts in the field.

Connecting with Communities and Experts:

Online Forums: Join online communities or forums where individuals share their experiences with breathing exercises. Websites like Reddit (r/Meditation and r/BreathingBuddies) and HealthBoards (healthboards.com) have active communities where you can ask questions, share insights, and connect with like-minded individuals.

Social Media: Follow experts, instructors, and organizations specializing in breathing exercises on social media platforms like Instagram, Facebook, and YouTube. Many experts regularly share tips, guided practices, and updates on research in the field.

Local Classes and Workshops: Check if there are local classes or workshops on breathing exercises and mindfulness in your area. Yoga studios, community centers, and senior centers often offer these classes. Attending in-person sessions can provide valuable guidance and a sense of community.

Consulting Experts: If you have specific health concerns or want personalized guidance, consider consulting experts such as respiratory therapists, yoga instructors, or mindfulness coaches. They can provide tailored recommendations based on your individual needs.

By exploring these additional resources, you can gain a deeper understanding of breathing exercises and respiratory health and connect with a supportive community of individuals who share your interests and goals. These resources will enhance your knowledge and help you make informed decisions on your path to better respiratory health and overall well-being.

Empowering Your Journey

As we conclude this comprehensive guide to breathing exercises and respiratory health for seniors, it's important to recognize the transformative power of knowledge and practice. You've embarked on a journey that can significantly enhance your overall well-being, and you now have a wealth of information at your fingertips to guide you along the way.

Empowerment Through Information: In today's world, access to reliable information is key to making informed decisions about your health. By delving into the chapters of this book, you've gained insights into the science, techniques, and benefits of breathing exercises. Armed with this knowledge, you have the tools to take control of your respiratory health and overall quality of life.

Final Words of Motivation

As we conclude this guide, let us emphasize that your journey with breathing exercises is a path filled with endless possibilities. The stories shared here are just a glimpse of what can be achieved through dedicated practice and an open heart.

With each conscious breath, you can nurture your physical health, sharpen your mental clarity, and embrace emotional balance. Remember that the benefits of these practices accumulate over time, and every breath you take is a step towards improved well-being.

So, dear reader, we leave you with this final message of motivation:

Your breath is a lifelong companion and a source of profound wisdom. Embrace it with curiosity, practice it with dedication, and experience the transformative power of Oxygen. As you continue exploring and practicing breathing exercises, you are investing in your own health, happiness, and vitality.

May your breath guide you towards a life of greater well-being and inner peace. The journey is yours to embrace, and the possibilities are limitless. Breathe deeply, live fully, and thrive in the golden years ahead.

MEET THE AUTHOR

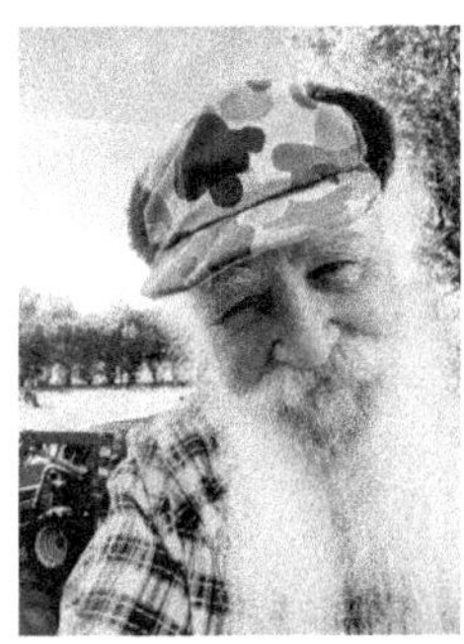 Jim Phillips, who holds a master's in education and has experience teaching graduate and undergraduate teachers, established, and ran two prominent educational institutions in the San Francisco Bay Area for 28 years. He founded Neighborhood Montessori, a well-known Early Childhood school, and The Gourmet Language School for Children, which gained recognition for its innovative foreign language programs in Spanish, French, Italian, and Mandarin Chinese, uniquely combined with culinary education. In 2006, after the big hurricane devastation, Jim, driven by his love for Louisiana, an extensive educational expertise and dedication to nurturing creativity in children, relocated to South Louisiana.

Jim Phillips shares his deep insights into the benefits of mastering breathing techniques. With over 55 years of personal experience, including teaching yoga in established centers in Columbia, MO, and Montreal, Canada, Jim illustrates the profound connection between body and mind through breathing exercises. He started his journey in the early 1970s, and the positive effects of various breathing techniques on his well-being motivated him to make them a part of his everyday life. His dedication to improving the lives of others through the power of breath is the driving force behind this book.

Jim invites readers to start their own journey of self-discovery. He offers practical advice and a wealth of knowledge gained over decades. For those seeking stress relief, better lung capacity, enhanced focus, preparation, or recovery from illness, or, even yet, a deeper connection with their own inner self, Jim's expertise in breathing exercises is an invaluable straightforward and easy to understand guide to holistic well-being.

9 798872 855729